50 Ways to Manage Type 2 Diabetes

Other books by M. Sara Rosenthal

The Thyroid Sourcebook
The Gynecological Sourcebook
The Pregnancy Sourcebook
The Fertility Sourcebook
The Breastfeeding Sourcebook
The Breast Sourcebook
The Gastrointestinal Sourcebook
Managing Your Diabetes
Managing Diabetes for Women
The Type 2 Diabetic Woman
The Thyroid Sourcebook for Women
Women & Sadness
Women & Depression
Women & Passion
Women of the '60s Turning 50
50 Ways to Prevent Colon Cancer
50 Ways Women Can Prevent Heart Disease
50 Ways to Relieve Heartburn, Reflux, and Ulcers

50 *Ways* to Manage Type 2 Diabetes

M. Sara Rosenthal

Foreword by
James McSherry, M.D., Ch.B.
Professor of Family Medicine,
University of Western Ontario,
Chief of Family Medicine
London Health Services Centre

Contemporary Books

Chicago   New York   San Francisco   Lisbon   London   Madrid   Mexico City
Milan   New Delhi   San Juan   Seoul   Singapore   Sydney   Toronto

Library of Congress Cataloging-in-Publication Data

Rosenthal, M. Sara.
    50 Ways to manage Type 2 diabetes / M. Sara Rosenthal.
       p.   cm.
    Includes bibliographical references and index.
    ISBN 0-7373-0540-1
      1. Non-insulin-dependent diabetes—Popular works.   I. Title: Fifty
    ways to manage Type 2 diabetes. II. Title

RC662.18 .R657   2001
616.4'62—dc21   00-066002

Contemporary Books

A Division of The McGraw·Hill Companies

  3 4 5 6 7 8 9 DOC/DOC 0 9 8 7 6 5

International Standard Book Number: 0-7373-0540-1

This book was set in Adobe Cochin and Abobe Futura by Jack Lanning
Printed and bound by R. R. Donnelley & Sons Co.

Cover design by Cheryl Carrington

McGraw-Hill books are available at special quantity discounts to use as premiums and sales promotions, or for use in corporate training programs. For more information, please write to the Director of Special Sales, Professional Publishing, McGraw-Hill, Two Penn Plaza, New York, NY 10121-2298. Or contact your local bookstore.

The purpose of this book is to educate. It is sold with the understanding that the publisher and author shall have neither liability nor responsibility for any injury caused or alleged to be caused directly or indirectly by the information contained in this book. While every effort has been made to ensure its accuracy, the book's contents should not be construed as medical advice. Each person's health needs are unique. To obtain recommendations appropriate to your particular situation, please consult a qualified health care provider.

This book is printed on acid-free paper.

Contents

Foreword

50 Ways to Manage Type 2 Diabetes is a timely book indeed. Demographic trends tell us that the number of Americans with Type 2 diabetes is going to increase dramatically over the next decade as the baby boomers move into middle age and beyond. Fortunately, there have been important developments in the management of Type 2 diabetes during the past several years, and it is now clear that the serious complications of diabetes are potentially avoidable, or at least treatable in a way that was impossible only a short time ago.

Surveys tell us that 95 percent of North Americans consult family physicians as their preferred point of entry into the health care system. About 80 percent of Americans with Type 2 diabetes receive medical care from their family physicians rather than specialists, and those figures are likely to increase as the scope of specialist practice changes. Family physicians, working as important members of a diabetes care team that includes nurses, diabetes educators, pharmacists, and other health professionals, have already begun to prepare themselves for greater responsibilities in the care of patients with diabetes.

With scientific advances, and likely changes in how medical care is going to be organized, has come the realization that diabetic care begins with the diabetic patient. The well-informed person with diabetes is his or her own biggest asset in dealing with a disease that has potentially serious consequences. It is surely no secret that doctors can't look after patients who don't—or won't—look after themselves.

The next best resource is a well-informed and interested family physician who is not only knowledgeable about diabetes, but who is proactive in organizing medical care by scheduling routine examinations, performing screening procedures for complications, and notifying patients with diabetes when annual influenza immunizations are due.

Sara Rosenthal is to be commended for writing this book. I sincerely hope that it will help Americans with diabetes increase their knowledge, develop new skills, and come to a fresh awareness of what they can do to help themselves.

—JAMES MCSHERRY, M.D., CH.B.,
Professor of Family Medicine,
University of Western Ontario,
Chief of Family Medicine London Health Services Centre

Introduction

What Is Type 2 Diabetes?

By 2004, one in four North Americans over the age of forty-five will be diagnosed with Type 2 diabetes. Whether you've just been diagnosed, or have been living with it for years, this is a difficult disease to understand. In fact, it is the most complicated condition I've ever written about, and I've tackled some tough health topics, including AIDS and cancer.

Why is Type 2 diabetes so hard to comprehend? Part of the problem is that there are so many names for this one disease, as there are for another type of diabetes, Type 1, so it's easy to lose track of what kind of diabetes you have. Clearing up this confusion is the first step in managing Type 2 diabetes, so let's begin by defining names and labels. Diabetes wasn't officially labeled Type 1 and Type 2 until 1979.

Type 2 diabetes means that your pancreas is functioning, and you are making plenty of insulin. In fact, you are probably making too much insulin, a condition called hyperinsulinemia ("too much insulin"). Insulin is a hormone made by your beta cells, the insulin-producing cells within the islets of Langerhans—small islands of cells afloat in your pancreas. The pancreas is a bird beak–shaped gland situated behind the stomach.

Insulin is a major player in our bodies. One of its most important functions is to regulate blood sugar levels. It does this by acting as a sort of courier, knocking on the cell's door, and announcing, "Sugar's here; come and get it!" Your cells then open the door to let sugar in from your bloodstream. That sugar is absolutely vital to your health and provides you with the energy you need to function.

But what happens if the cells don't answer the door? Two things. First, the sugar in your bloodstream will accumulate, having nowhere to go. It's like having your newspapers pile up outside your front door when you're away. Second, your pancreas will keep sending out more couriers to try to get your cells to open that door and take in the "newspapers." The result of the cells' not complying is a pile of newspapers and a lineup of unsuccessful couriers by your door. When the cell doesn't answer the door, this is called insulin resistance; the cell is resisting insulin. The end result is diabetes, which means "high blood sugar." A synonym for diabetes is hyperglycemia, which also means "high blood sugar." If insulin resistance goes on for too long, the pancreas can become overworked and eventually may not make enough, or any, insulin. In effect, it's like a courier strike. And finally, the liver, being the good neighbor that it is, will lend a bowl or two of sugar to the sugar-deprived cell. But this can exacerbate existing high blood sugar.

Type 2 diabetes, a genetic disease, is a completely different illness than Type 1 diabetes, an autoimmune disease.

Type 1 diabetes is also known as juvenile diabetes or insulin-dependent diabetes mellitus (IDDM). Only 10 percent of all people with diabetes have Type 1 diabetes. Type 2 diabetes, on the other hand, accounts for 90 percent of all those with diabetes. Since Type 2 diabetes doesn't usually develop until after age forty-five, it was once known as mature-onset diabetes or adult-onset diabetes. And since Type 2 diabetes is a disease of insulin resistance, rather than no insulin, it often can be managed through diet and exercise, without insulin injections. For this reason, Type 2 diabetes was also known as non-insulin-dependent diabetes mellitus (NIDDM). All these labels have been replaced by the term *Type 2 diabetes*.

Here's where it gets really confusing! When you are told that you have "non-insulin-dependent diabetes," it doesn't mean that you will never require insulin. Insulin resistance, characterized by the body's inability to use insulin, sometimes leads to a condition in which the pancreas stops making insulin altogether. The cells' resistance to insulin causes the pancreas to work harder, causing too much insulin in the system (hyperinsulinemia) until it just plumb tuckers out, as the saying goes. Your pancreas is making the insulin and knocking on the door, but the cells aren't answering. Your pancreas will eventually say, "Okay, fine! I'll shut down production, since you obviously aren't using what I'm making." A lot of people with Type 2 diabetes confuse requiring insulin with Type 1 diabetes, falsely believing that their Type 2 diabetes has turned into Type 1. Type 2 diabetes cannot turn into Type 1 diabetes any more than an apple can turn into a banana. So what do you call it when someone with Type 2 diabetes requires insulin? This is known as insulin-requiring Type 2 diabetes. In fact, about one-third of all people with Type 2 diabetes will eventually need insulin therapy.

Something else you need to understand about Type 2 diabetes is that the high blood sugar that results from insulin resistance can lead to a number of other diseases, including cardiovascular disease (heart disease and stroke) and peripheral vascular disease (PVD), in which blood doesn't flow properly to other parts of the body. This can create a number of problems; these are discussed under Preventing Complications. Many people who suffer a heart attack or stroke have Type 2 diabetes.

Roughly 6 percent of all Caucasian adults have Type 2 diabetes, but the disease affects African North Americans at a rate of 12 to 15 percent, Latinos at a rate of 20 percent, and Native North Americans at a rate exceeding 30 percent. In some Native communities, up to 70 percent of adults have Type 2 diabetes. Your goal in managing Type 2 diabetes is to control your blood sugar levels and weight through diet and exercise and to prevent long-term complications of the disease. The first step in controlling your diabetes is eliminating your diabetes symptoms and remaining as symptom free as possible. Meal planning combined with exercise is the best way to do this. These strategies will help you lose weight if needed as well as distribute an even amount of calories to your body throughout the day. If you don't put any unusual strain on your body's metabolism, you will likely not experience any surprises when it comes to your blood sugar levels. Exercise makes insulin much more available to your cells, while your muscles use sugar as fuel.

If you have been diagnosed with Type 2 diabetes, the good news is that you are living at a time when self-managing your diabetes has never been easier. There are not only brand-new treatment options available, but also dozens of upgraded products to make your diabetes a lot easier to monitor. The bad news is that only you can manage your diabetes. This is one of those diseases that can't be controlled only by your doctor. You have to take charge, while your doctor supervises from afar. For this reason, being diagnosed with diabetes may feel like being pushed out of an airplane without a parachute. Think of this book as basic training: It will tell you what you need to know to plan for a safe landing. It will also serve as a user's guide to diabetes equipment: glucose monitors (optional), pills, and, in some cases, insulin and all its gear.

PART ONE

Controlling Blood Sugar

1. Understand Normal Versus High Blood Sugar

Knowing the symptoms of both high and low blood sugar is crucial when you're trying to manage Type 2 diabetes. All the following symptoms could be signs of high blood sugar, also called hyperglycemia or diabetes:

- Weight gain. When your body is not using insulin properly, you may suffer from excess insulin, which can increase your appetite. This is a classic Type 2 symptom.

- Blurred vision or any change in sight. You may feel that your prescription eyewear has become weak.

- Drowsiness or extreme fatigue at times when you shouldn't be drowsy or tired.

- Frequent infections that are slow to heal. (Women should be on alert for recurring vaginal yeast infections or vaginitis, which means vaginal inflammation, characterized by itching and/or foul-smelling discharge.)

- Tingling or numbness in the hands and feet.
- Gum disease. High blood sugar affects the blood vessels in your mouth, causing inflamed gums; the sugar content can get into your saliva, causing cavities in your teeth.

Diabetes experts point out that the following may also be signs of Type 2 diabetes:

- Irregular periods in women, such as changes in cycle length or flow. (This could be a sign of menopause as well.)
- Depression, which could be a symptom of either low or high blood sugar.
- Headaches (from hypoglycemia).
- Insomnia and/or nightmares (from hypoglycemia).
- Spots on the shin (known as necrobiosis diabeticorum).
- Decaying toenails.
- Muscle pains or aches after exercise. (High blood sugar can cause lactic acid to build up, which can cause pain that prevents you from continuing exercise.)

You may also have diabetes if your doctor has diagnosed you with the following:

- High cholesterol.
- High blood pressure.
- Anemia.
- Cataracts.
- Salivary-gland stones.

Early signs of high blood sugar are extreme thirst, dry and flushed skin, mood swings, or unusual fatigue—but many people notice no symptoms at all.

One thing you don't need to worry about, however, is forming ketones (ketone bodies)—poisonous chemicals the body manufactures in desperation as a source of energy when no glucose is available. In people with Type 1 diabetes, high ketones along with high blood sugar cause diabetic ketoacidosis (DKA), which is an emergency situation. Signs of DKA include frequent urination (polyuria), excessive thirst (polydipsia), excessive hunger (polyphagia), and a fruity smell to the breath. But people with Type 2 diabetes do not form ketones. That's because the cells never think they are starving, since insulin still comes to knock at the door and the liver continues to make glucose.

Understanding the Numbers

Before September 1998, many people with Type 2 diabetes were told they had impaired glucose tolerance (IGT), which was more widely known as borderline diabetes. For the record, there is no such thing as borderline diabetes. But in light of new guidelines announced in 1998, many people once diagnosed with IGT will now be diagnosed with diabetes.

IGT was what many doctors referred to as the "gray zone" between normal blood sugar levels and full-blown diabetes. Normal fasting blood sugar levels (what they are before you've eaten) are between 60 milligrams per deciliter (mg/dl) and 90 mg/dl (or, on the metric system, 3.3 to 5.0 millimoles per liter—mmol/L). To convert "mg/dl" to "mmol/L" simply divide by 18; you may need to know this if you're traveling in Canada or Europe, for example.

In the past, three fasting blood glucose levels between 90 mg/dl (5.0 mmol/L) and 140 mg/dl (7.8 mmol/L) meant that a person had IGT. A fasting blood glucose level over 140 mg/dl (7.8 mmol/L) or a random (any time of day) blood glucose level greater than 200 mg/dl (or 11.1 mmol/L) meant that a person had diabetes.

But that's all changed. Today, anyone with a fasting blood sugar level higher than 126 mg/dl (7.0 mmol/L) is considered to be in the diabetic range and is officially diagnosed with Type 2 diabetes. A new term has also been introduced, impaired fasting glucose (IFG), which refers to blood glucose levels between 110 mg/dl and less than 126 mg/dl (6.1 mmol/L and 7.0 mmol/L). The term *IGT* is now used only when describing people who have a blood glucose level between 140 mg/dl and 200 mg/dl (7.8 mmol/L and 11.1 mmol/L) two hours after an oral glucose tolerance test. See Table 1.1 for more details.

If you can't seem to keep your fasting blood sugar levels below 126 mg/dl (7.0 mmol/L), you are probably a candidate for an antidiabetes pill or an oral hypoglycemic pill, discussed in Part Four.

TABLE 1.1 What Your Blood Sugar Readings Mean

	Fasting:	
Normal	**IFG***	**Diabetes**
<110 mg/dl	>110 mg/dl to	>126 mg/dl (7.0)
(6.1 mmol/L)	<126 mg/dl	
	(>6.1 mmol/L to <7.0 mmol/L)	

	Two hours after an oral glucosetolerance test:	
Normal	**IGT****	**Diabetes**
<140 mg/dl	>140 mg/dl	>200 mg/dl
(7.8 mmol/L)	to <200 mg/dl	(11.1 mmol/L)
	(>7.8 mmol/L to <11.1 mmol/L)	

* IFG stands for impaired fasting glucose.
** IGT stands for impaired glucose tolerance, referring to test results two hours after an oral glucose tolerance test.

Syndrome X

Also known as the metabolic syndrome, the name Syndrome X was coined by Dr. Gerald Reaven, professor of medicine at Stanford University. It describes a condition characterized by high blood insulin levels and an elevated risk of heart disease. This is indistinguishable from IGT, but Dr. Reaven insists that people with Syndrome X do not generally develop full-blown Type 2 diabetes. The problem here is that the high insulin levels can still predispose you to risk factors for cardiovascular problems. Dr. Reaven's research showed that a high-carbohydrate diet could raise insulin levels and blood pressure in people with Syndrome X. The myth about Syndrome X is that it causes obesity, which Reaven states is untrue.

Nonetheless, Syndrome X has now fueled a whole industry of diet books promoting low- or no-carbohydrate diets, such as *Dr. Atkins' New Diet Revolution*, *Protein Power*, and *The Zone*. The diets promoted in these books, however, are considered by Dr. Reaven and other diabetes experts to be dangerous to anyone with Syndrome X, IGT, and especially Type 2 diabetes. The Dr. Atkins plan is dangerous because it is based on a huge amount of saturated fat, which is the major source of LDL (low-density lipoprotein) or "bad cholesterol" in the diet. People with Syndrome X tend to have higher bad cholesterol levels, as well as a reduced ability to break up blood clots. Regardless of how much weight you may lose on the Atkins diet, you are still at risk for heart disease because of the saturated fat and high LDL levels. The Zone diet, according to Reaven, has no scientific basis; the book claims that high carbs and insulin make you fat, when in fact, calories from all sources of food can make you fat if you don't burn them off through physical activity.

The best advice if you have Syndrome X is to limit your carbohydrates to 45 percent of calories. On a 2000-calorie per day diet, this would be roughly 225 grams of carbohydrates per day. For more information on meal planning, see Items 21 through 30.

2. Buy a Glucose Meter and Test Your Blood Sugar

All diabetes experts agree that the most important way to begin to control your blood sugar is to purchase a glucose meter and test your blood sugar about three or four times a day. In a newly diagnosed person with Type 2 diabetes, frequent daily testing will show individual patterns of glucose rises and dips. This information may help your health care team tailor your meal plans, exercise routines, and medication regimens. And if you do have to take insulin in the future, you will need to get into the habit of testing your own blood sugar anyway. (By getting your diet under control, you can avoid requiring insulin.)

As in the computer industry, glucose meter manufacturers tend to come out with technological upgrades every year. In fact, you can now purchase systems that download the time, date, and blood sugar values for the last 125 glucose tests right onto your personal computer. This information can help you gauge whether your diet and exercise routine are working, or whether you need to adjust your medications or insulin. All glucose monitors provide the following:

- A battery-powered, pocket-sized device.
- An LED screen (that is, a calculatorlike screen).
- Accurate results in thirty to sixty seconds.

- The date and time of your test result.
- A recall memory of at least your last ten readings.
- At least a one-year warranty.
- The opportunity to upgrade.
- A toll-free customer service hotline.
- Mailings and giveaways every so often.
- A few free lancets (to prick your finger) with your purchase; you may have to separately buy what's known as a lancing device, a sort of Pez dispenser for your lancets. (Eventually, you'll run out of lancets and have to buy those, too.)

No matter which glucose meter you choose, these instructions can serve as a general guideline:

- Before testing, wash your hands with an antibacterial soap.
- Pierce your finger on the side rather than top, and obtain a hanging drop of blood (some newer devices suck out your blood for you).
- Smear or blot your drop of blood onto a plastic strip that looks like a strip of tape without the sticky side. (Whether you smear or wipe depends on your glucose meter.)
- Turn on your glucose meter and place the strip into the machine.
- The results will show up on the calculatorlike screen.
- Record these results in a logbook. Hint: A good result before meals ranges from 72 to 126 mg/dl (4 to 7 mmol/L); a good result after meals ranges from 90 to 180 mg/dl (5 to 10 mmol/L).

Tainted Results

Most people are not testing their blood sugar under squeaky-clean laboratory conditions. The following outside factors may interfere with your meter's performance:

- Other medications you're taking. Studies show that some meters can be inaccurate if you're taking acetaminophen, salicylate, ascorbic acid, dopamine, or levodopa. As a rule, if you're taking any medications, check with your doctor, pharmacist, and glucose meter manufacturer (call the toll-free number) about whether your drugs can affect the meter's accuracy.

- Humidity. The worst place to keep your meter and strips is in the bathroom where humidity can ruin the strips, unless they're individually wrapped in foil. Keep strips in a sealed container away from extreme temperatures. Use videotape rules; for example, don't store your meter and strips in a car's hot glove compartment. Don't keep them in the freezer, either.

- Bright light. Ever tried to use a calculator or portable computer in bright sunlight? It's not possible because the light interferes with the screen. Some meters are photometric, which means they are affected by bright light. If you plan to test in sunlight, get a biosenser meter that is unaffected by bright light (there are several).

- Touching the test strip. Many glucose meters come with test strips that cannot be touched with your fingers or a second drop of blood. If you're all thumbs, purchase a meter that is unaffected by touch and/or allows a second drop of blood.

- **Wet hands.** Before you test, thoroughly dry your hands. Water can dilute your blood sample.
- **Motion.** It's always best to test yourself when you're standing still. Testing on planes, trains, automobiles, buses, and subways may affect your results, depending on the brand of glucose meter.
- **Dirt, lint, and blood.** Particles of dirt, lint, and old blood can sometimes affect the accuracy of a meter, depending on the brand. Make sure you clean the meter regularly (follow the manufacturer's cleaning directions) to remove buildup. Make sure you change the batteries, too! There are meters on the market that do not require cleaning and are unaffected by dirt, but they may cost a little more.

3. Know When to Test Your Blood Sugar

In the days when diabetes patients went to their doctors' offices for blood sugar testing, they were usually tested first thing in the morning before eating (called a fasting blood sugar level) or immediately after eating (known as a postprandial or postmeal blood sugar level). It was believed that if either the fasting or postprandial levels were normal, the patient was stable. This is now known to be completely false. In fact, your blood sugar levels can bounce around all day long. Because your blood sugar is constantly changing, a blood sugar test in a doctor's office is pretty useless; it measures what your blood sugar is only for that nanosecond. In other words, what your blood sugar is at 2:15 P.M. is not what it might be at 3:05 P.M.

It makes the most sense to test yourself before each meal, so you know what your levels are before you eat anything, as well as about two hours after meals. Immediately after eating, everybody's blood sugar is high, so this is not the ideal time for anyone to test. In a person without diabetes, blood sugar levels drop about two hours after eating in response to the natural insulin the body makes. Therefore, you should test yourself two hours after eating to make sure that you are able to "mimic" a normal blood sugar pattern, too. Ideally, this translates into at least four blood tests daily:

1. When you wake up.
2. After breakfast/before lunch (two hours after breakfast).
3. After lunch/before dinner (two hours after lunch).
4. After dinner or at bedtime (two hours after dinner).

It's also important to know the answers to these questions:

- What is your blood sugar level as soon as you wake up? (It should be at its lowest point.)
- What is your blood sugar level two hours after a meal? (It should be much lower two hours after eating than one hour after eating.)
- What is your blood sugar level when you feel ill? (You need to avoid dipping too low or high since your routine is changing.)

4. Request a Glycosylated Hemoglobin Test

This most important test checks your glycosylated hemoglobin levels (the glucose attached to the protein in your red blood cells) and is known as the hemoglobin A1c test or the HbA1c test. Hemoglobin is a large molecule that carries oxygen to the bloodstream. When the glucose in your blood comes in contact with the hemoglobin molecule, it conveniently sticks to it. The more glucose stuck to your hemoglobin, the higher your blood sugar is. The HbA1c test measures the amount of glucose stuck to hemoglobin. And since each hemoglobin molecule stays in your blood about three to four months before it is replaced, this test can show you the average blood sugar level over the last three to four months. Therefore, this test is recommended at least every six months. If you have cardiovascular problems, you will need to have the HbA1c test more often.

A similar test, known as a fructosamine test, can show the amount of glucose stuck to a molecule in your blood known as albumin. Albumin, however, gets replaced every four to six weeks, so this test can therefore give you an average of blood sugar levels only over the last four to six weeks.

What's a Good HbA1c Result?

Just like your glucose monitor at home, the goal of the HbA1c test is to make sure that your blood sugar average is as close to normal as possible. Again, the closer to normal it is, the less likely you are to experience long-term diabetes complications.

This test result is slightly different than your glucose meter result. For example, an HbA1c level of 7.0 percent is equal to 144 mg/dl (8 mmol/L) on your blood glucose meter. A result of 9.5 percent is equivalent to 234 mg/dl (13 mmol/L) on your blood glucose meter. In a person without diabetes, an HbA1c ranges from 4 to 6 percent. The results are often expressed as percentages of "normal," such as <110 percent, 111–140 percent, or >140 percent.

The new guidelines stipulate that values of 6 percent or less are good results and mean that your blood sugar is perfectly under control. Meanwhile, anything higher than 8.4 percent is alarming; this would be a poor result and means that your diabetes is out of control. Studies show that when your HbA1c result is 8.4 percent or higher, you have a greater chance of developing long-term complications. In fact, for every 10 percent drop in your HbA1c average (that is, 7.1 percent down from 8.1 percent), the risk of long-term complications falls by about 40 percent. (See Table 4.1 for guidelines.)

Problems with the HbA1c Test

If your child came home from school with a report card showing a B average, it doesn't mean your child is getting a B in every course; it means that he or she could have received a D in one course and an A+ in another. Similarly, the HbA1c test is just an average mark. You could have a decent result, even though your blood sugar levels may be dangerously low one day and dangerously high the next.

If you suffer from sickle-cell disease or other blood disorders, the HbA1c results will not be accurate, either. In this case, you may wind up with either false high or low readings.

TABLE 4.1 What's a Good Glycosylated Hemoglobin Test (HbA1c) Result?

	Range		
Nondiabetic	**Optimal**	**Suboptimal**	**Poor Control**
4–6.0%	<7.0%	7.0–8.4%	>8.4%
	<100–115%	116–140%	>140%

If at any time your home blood sugar tests (if you've opted for self-testing) over the past two or three months do not seem to match the results of the HbA1c test, be sure to check the accuracy of your meter, and perhaps show your doctor or certified diabetes educator how you are using the meter, in case your technique needs some refining.

5. Start a Health Diary

All the information you're collecting in Items 1, 2, and 3 should be the basis for a health diary, which you share with your doctor or diabetes health care provider. The most important information your health diary will contain is the pattern of your blood sugar's peaks and valleys. Dates and times of these peaks and valleys may be important clues for establishing your pattern. Your meal plan, exercise routine, and medication regimen should be tailored to anticipate these peaks and valleys. You may need to incorporate a snack to prevent a low, or go for a twenty-minute walk after dinner to prevent a high. Since there are a variety of factors that can affect your blood sugar levels, your diary should also record:

- Any medication you're taking.
- Unusually high or low readings that fall outside your pattern.
- Stressful life events or situations.
- Illness.
- Out-of-the-ordinary happenings (no matter how insignificant).
- Changes in your health insurance or status.

- Severe insulin reactions (if you're taking insulin).
- General medical history (for example, surgeries, tests you've had done, allergies, past drug reactions).

6. Learn to Prevent High Blood Sugar

Common reasons for a change in blood sugar levels revolve around the following:

- Overeating or eating more than usual.
- A change in exercise routine.
- Missing a medication dose or an insulin shot (if you're taking insulin).
- An out-of-the-ordinary event (illness, stress, upset, excitement).
- A sudden mood change (extreme fright, anger, or sadness).
- Pregnancy.

In response to unusual strains or stress, your body taps into its stored glucose supplies for extra energy. This raises your blood sugar level as more glucose than normal is released into your system. Whether you're fighting off a flu or fighting with your mother, digesting all the food you ate at that all-you-can-eat buffet, or running away from a black bear, your body will try to give you the extra boost of energy you need to get through your immediate crisis.

Blood sugar levels naturally rise when you're ill. In the event of a cold, fever, flu, or injury, you'll need to adjust your routine to accommodate high blood sugar levels, especially if vomiting or diarrhea is occurring. In some cases, you may need to go on insulin temporarily. When you're ill and you have Type 2 diabetes, it's crucial to see your doctor.

7. Learn to Prevent Low Blood Sugar

When you're diagnosed with Type 2 diabetes, whether your treatment revolves around lifestyle modification, oral hypoglycemic drugs, or insulin therapy, you may experience an episode of low blood sugar. Hypoglycemia can sometimes come on suddenly, particularly overnight. Planning your meals around your activity should prevent episodes of low blood sugar.

Any blood sugar reading below 70 mg/dl (3.8 mmol/L) is considered too low. A hypoglycemic episode is characterized by two stages: the warning stage and what I call the actual hypoglycemic episode. The warning stage occurs when your blood sugar levels begin to drop and can occur as early as a blood sugar reading of 108 mg/dl (6.0 mmol/L), in people with typically higher-than-normal blood sugar levels. When your blood sugar drops to below 55 mg/dl (or 3.0 mmol/L), you are officially hypoglycemic.

If you can begin to recognize the warning signs of hypoglycemia (see below and Item 8), you may be able to stabilize your blood sugar before you lose consciousness. Most people will feel hungry and headachy, then sweaty, nervous, and dizzy. Those who live with or spend a lot of time with you should learn to notice sudden mood changes (usually extreme irritability, drunklike aggression, and confusion) as a warning that you are low. Whether you notice your own mood changes or not, you, too, will feel suddenly unwell. By simply asking yourself, "Why is this happening?," you should be able to remember that it's a warning that your blood sugar is low and reach for your snack pack (see Item 9). The irritability can simulate the ranting of someone who is drunk, while the weakness and shakiness can lead to the lack of coordination seen in someone who is drunk. For this reason, it's crucial that you carry a card or wear a bracelet that identifies you as having diabetes. If left untreated, hypoglycemia can result in coma, brain damage, and death. Hypoglycemia is considered the official cause of death in about 5 percent of the Type 1 diabetic population; and in the past, hypoglycemia was more common among people with Type 1 diabetes than those with Type 2. But since 40 to 50 percent of all people with Type 2 diabetes will eventually graduate to insulin therapy, the incidence of hypoglycemia has increased by 300 percent in this group. Moreover, hypoglycemia is a common side effect of oral hypoglycemic pills (see Item 32), the medication the majority of people with Type 2 take when they are first diagnosed.

An episode of hypoglycemia can be triggered by:

- Delaying or missing a meal or snack. (See Item 21.)
- Drinking alcohol. (See Item 27.)
- Exercising too long or strong without compensating with extra food. (See Item 13.)
- Taking too high a dose of an oral hypoglycemic agent. (This can happen if you lose weight but are not put on a lower dose of your pill. See Item 32.)

Low blood sugar can also be the result of too high an insulin dose, which is what is meant by the term *insulin shock* (or insulin reaction). This is a misleading term, however, because it implies that only people who take insulin can become hypoglycemic.

If You're Taking Pills

About 15 to 30 percent of all people taking sulphonylureas (see Part Four) are vulnerable to hypoglycemia because these drugs stimulate the pancreas to produce insulin. This is the same as taking an insulin injection. If you lose weight after you begin taking sulphonylureas, but don't lower your pill dosage, you could also experience hypoglycemic episodes because weight loss makes your body more responsive to insulin.

8. Know How to Handle an Episode of Low Blood Sugar

No one with diabetes is immune to hypoglycemia; it can occur in a person with long-standing diabetes just as easily as in someone newly diagnosed. The important thing is to be alert to the warning signs. Not everyone experiences the same warning symptoms, but here are some signs to watch for:

- Pounding, racing heart.
- Breathing fast.
- Skin turning white.
- Sweating (cold sweat in big drops).
- Trembling, tremors, or shaking.
- Goose bumps or pale, cool skin.
- Extreme hunger pangs.
- Light-headedness (feeling dizzy or that the room is spinning).
- Nervousness, extreme irritability, or a sudden mood change.
- Confusion.
- Feeling weak or faint.
- Headache.
- Vision changes (seeing double or blurry vision).

Some people experience no symptoms at all. If you've had a hypoglycemic episode without any warning signs, it's important for you to eat regularly and to test your blood sugar. If you're experiencing frequent hypoglycemic episodes, diabetes educators recommend that by keeping your sugar above normal, you can prevent low blood sugar. In some cases of long-standing diabetes and repeated hypoglycemic episodes, experts note that the warning symptoms may not always occur. It's believed that in some people, the body eventually loses its ability to detect hypoglycemia and send out adrenaline. Furthermore, if you've switched from animal to human insulin, warning symptoms may not be as pronounced.

If you start to feel symptoms of hypoglycemia, stop what you're doing (especially if it's active) and have some sugar. Next, test your blood sugar to see what it reads. Regular food will usually do the trick. If your blood sugar is below 70 mg/dl (3.8 mmol/L), ingest some glucose or simple sugar; that is, sugar that gets into your bloodstream quickly. Half a cup of any fruit juice or one-third a can of a sugary soft drink is a good source of simple sugar. Artificially sweetened soft drinks are useless; it must be real sugar. If you don't have fruit juice or soft drinks handy, here are some other sources of simple sugar:

- Two to three tablets of commercial dextrose, sold in pharmacies. If you're taking acarbose or combining it with an oral hypoglycemic agent or insulin, the only sugar you can have is dextrose (Dextrosol or Monoject), due to the rate of absorption.

- Three to five hard candies. (That's equal to about six LifeSavers.)

- Two teaspoons of white or brown sugar (or two sugar cubes).
- One tablespoon of honey.

Once you've ingested enough simple sugar, your hypoglycemic symptoms should disappear within ten to fifteen minutes. Test your blood sugar ten minutes after eating sugar to see if your blood sugar levels are coming back up. If your symptoms don't go away, ingest more simple sugars until they do.

9. Keep a Snack Pack Handy

You can avoid sugar swings by keeping a snack pack with you for emergencies or for unplanned physical activity. The pack should contain:

- Juice (two to three boxes or cans).
- Sweet soft drinks — sweetened with real sugar, not sugar substitutes (two cans).
- A bag of hard candies.
- Some protein and carbohydrates (for example, packaged cheese and crackers).
- Granola bars (great for after exercise).
- A card that reads "I have diabetes."

10. Have These Things Checked Regularly

It's important to have the following routine tests performed at least once a year, and more often if you are at high risk for complications.

Glucose Meter Checkup

If you've opted to test your own blood sugar, it's important to compare your home glucose meter's test results to a laboratory blood glucose test. In fact, it's a good idea to do this every six months. Bring your meter to the lab when you're having a blood glucose test done. After the lab technician takes your blood, do your own test within about five minutes and record the result. Your meter is working perfectly so long as your result is within 15 percent of the lab test result (if your meter is testing whole blood, as opposed to plasma).

Blood Pressure

High blood pressure can put you at greater risk for cardiovascular problems. Diabetes can also cause high blood pressure. That's why it's important to have your blood pressure checked every four to six months. Blood pressure is measured in two readings: X over Y. The X is the systolic pressure, which is the pressure that occurs during the heart's contraction. The Y is the diastolic pressure, which is the pressure that occurs when the heart rests between contractions. Think of your heart as a liquid-soap hand pump: the systolic pressure occurs when you press the pump down; the diastolic pressure occurs when you release the pump and allow it to return to its resting position.

Normal blood pressure readings are 120 over 80 (120/80). Readings of 140/90 or higher are generally considered borderline, although for some people this is still considered a normal reading. For the general population, 140/90 is "lecture time," when your doctor will counsel you about dietary and lifestyle habits. By 160/100, many people are prescribed an anti-hypertensive drug, which is designed to lower blood pressure.

Kidney Tests

One of the most common complications of diabetes is kidney disease, known in this case as diabetic nephropathy (diabetic kidney disease). This condition develops slowly over the course of many years, but there are usually few symptoms or warning signs. To make sure no damage to the kidneys has occurred, it's important to have your urine tested regularly to check the health of your kidneys.

Cholesterol

Diabetes can trigger high cholesterol. Your cholesterol is checked through a simple blood test that should be done once on diagnosis, and once a year thereafter. Table 10.1 shows cholesterol level readings and their risk.

TABLE 10.1 Lipid Levels

Cholesterol Levels

<200 mg/dl (11.11 mmol/L)	Desirable
200–239 mg/dl (11.11–13.28 mmol/L)	Borderline
>240 mg/dl (13.33 mmol/L)	High

Low-Density Lipoprotein Levels

<130 mg/dl (7.22 mmol/L)	Desirable
130–159 mg/dl (7.22–8.83 mmol/L)	Borderline
>160 mg/dl (8.88 mmol/L)	High

High-Density Lipoprotein Levels

>35 mg/dl (1.9 mmol/L)	Desirable

Foot Exam

When you have diabetes, nerve damage and poor circulation can wreak havoc on your feet. Be sure to have a thorough foot exam each year to check for reduced sensation or feeling, circulation, evidence of calluses, or sores. (See Item 48 for more details.)

Eye Exam

Since diabetes can cause what's known as diabetes eye disease or diabetic retinopathy (damage to the back of the eye), annual eye exams are crucial. Your eye exam should also rule out cataracts and glaucoma. When caught early, laser treatment can be used to treat diabetic eye disease and prevent blindness. If your exam results record the term *absent* on your chart, it means your retina is just fine. If you see the term *background*, it means that mild changes have occurred to your eye(s) and that you need more regular monitoring. If the terms *preproliferative* or *proliferative* are used, there is some damage to one or both eyes, and you will require treatment and regular exams. (See Item 47 for more details.)

PART TWO

Active Living

11. Understand What Exercise Really Means

The *Oxford English Dictionary* defines exercise as "the exertion of muscles, limbs, etc., especially for health's sake; bodily, mental, or spiritual training." In the Western world, we have placed an emphasis on bodily training when we talk about exercise, completely ignoring mental and spiritual training. Only recently have Western studies begun to focus on the mental benefits of exercise. (It's been shown, for example, that exercise creates endorphins, hormones that make us feel good.) But we in the West do not encourage meditation or other calming forms of mental and spiritual exercise, which have also been shown to improve well-being and health, particularly in reducing stress—a major risk factor for heart disease.

In the East, for thousands of years, exercise has focused on achieving mental and spiritual health through the body, using breathing and postures, for example. Fitness practitioner Karen Faye maintains that posture is extremely important for organ alignment. Standing correctly, with ears over shoulders and shoulders over hips, with knees slightly bent and head straight up, naturally allows you to pull in your abdomen. According to Faye, many native cultures in which people balance baskets over their heads or do a lot of physical work with their bodies are noted for correct postures and low rates of osteoporosis.

Nor should we ignore cultural traditions known to improve mental health and well-being, such as traditional dances, active prayers that incorporate physical activity, circles that involve community and communication, and sweat lodges, believed to help rid the body of toxins through sweating. These are all forms of wellness activities that you should investigate.

12. Understand What Aerobic Means

If you look up the word *aerobic* in the dictionary, what you'll find is the chemical definition: "living in free oxygen." Humans are aerobes—beings that require oxygen to live. Some bacteria, however, are anaerobic; they can exist in an environment without oxygen.

When we exercise aerobically, we raise the oxygen level in our blood. All that jumping around and fast movement makes us breathe faster, so we can take more oxygen into our bodies. Why are we doing this? Because the blood contains oxygen! The faster your blood flows, the more oxygen can flow to your organs.

But when your health care practitioner tells you to exercise or to take up aerobic exercise, he or she is not referring solely to increasing oxygen but to exercising the heart muscle. The faster it beats, the better a workout it gets. If you already have heart disease or are on medications that affect your heart, check with your doctor to make sure you are not overworking your heart.

Why We Want More Oxygen

When more oxygen is in our bodies, we burn fat (see below), our breathing improves, our blood pressure improves, and our hearts work better. Oxygen also lowers triglycerides and cholesterol, increasing our high-density lipoproteins (HDL) or the "good cholesterol," while decreasing our low-density lipoproteins (LDL) or the "bad cholesterol." This means that your arteries will unclog, and you may significantly decrease your risk of heart disease and stroke. More oxygen makes our brains work better, so we feel better. Studies show that depression is decreased when we increase oxygen flow into our bodies. Ancient techniques such as yoga, which specifically improve mental and spiritual well-being, achieve this by combining deep breathing and stretching, which improves oxygen and blood flow to specific parts of the body.

Exercise has been shown to dramatically decrease the incidence of many other diseases, including cancer. Some research suggests that cancer cells tend to thrive in an oxygen-depleted environment. The more oxygen in the blood-stream, the less hospitable you make your body to cancer. In addition, since many cancers are related to fat-soluble toxins, the less fat on your body, the less fat-soluble toxins your body can accumulate.

Burning Fat

The only kind of exercise that will burn fat is aerobic exercise, because oxygen burns fat. If you were to go to your fridge and pull out some animal fat (chicken skin, red-meat fat, or butter), throw it in the sink, and light it with a match, it will burn. What makes the flame yellow is oxygen; what fuels the fire is the fat. That same process goes on in your body. The oxygen will burn your fat, no matter how you increase the oxygen flow in your body—by jumping around and increasing your heart rate or by using a deep-breathing technique (see Item 14).

The Western Definition of Aerobic

In the West, an exercise is considered aerobic if it makes your heart beat faster than it normally does. When your heart is beating fast, you'll be breathing hard and sweating and will ideally be in your "target zone" or "ideal range" (the kind of phrases that turn many people off).

There are official calculations you can do to find this target range. For example, if you subtract your age from 220, then multiply that number by 60 percent, you will find your threshold level—which means, "Your heart should be beating X beats per minute for twenty to thirty minutes." If you multiply the number by 75 percent, you will find your ceiling level—which means, "Your heart should not be beating faster than X beats per minute for twenty to thirty minutes." But this is only an example. If you are on heart medications (drugs that slow your heart down, known as beta blockers), you'll want to make sure you discuss what target to aim for with your health professional.

Finding Your Pulse

You have pulse points all over your body. The easiest ones to find are those on your neck, at the base of your thumb, just below your earlobe, and on your wrist. To check your heart rate, look at a watch or clock and begin to count your beats for fifteen seconds. Then multiply by 4 to get your pulse.

The Borg's Rate of Perceived Exertion (RPE)

The RPE or Borg scale measures exercise intensity without finding your pulse and, because of its simplicity, is now the recommended method for judging exertion. The scale goes from 6 to 20. Extremely light activity may rate a 7, for example, while a very, very hard activity may rate a 19. Exercise practitioners recommend that you do a talk test to rate your exertion, too. If you can't talk without gasping for air, you may be working too hard. You should be able to carry on a normal conversation throughout light to moderate activity. What's crucial to remember about RPE is that it is extremely individual; what one person judges a 7 another may judge to be a 10.

13. Understand the Muscle-Sugar Connection

Forty percent of your body weight is made from muscle, where sugar is stored. The muscles use this sugar when they are being worked. When the sugar is used up, the muscles, in a healthy body, will drink in sugar from the blood. After exercising, the muscles will continue to drink in glucose from the blood to replenish the glucose that was there before exercise.

But when you have insulin resistance, glucose from your blood has difficulty getting inside your muscles; the muscles act like a brick wall. As you begin to use and tone your muscles, they will become more receptive to the glucose in your blood, allowing the glucose in. Studies show that a muscle worked out in a given exercise takes up glucose far more easily than another muscle in the same person that has not been worked out.

Doing weight-bearing activities is also encouraged because these build bone mass and use up calories. Building bone mass is particularly important; as Karen Faye says, "If you want a strong house, you need a strong frame!" Women are vulnerable to osteoporosis (loss of bone mass) as a result of estrogen loss after menopause (unless they are on hormone replacement therapy) and will especially benefit from these activities. The denser your bones, the harder they are to break. As we age, we are all at risk for osteoporosis unless we've either been building up our bone mass for years or are maintaining our current bone mass.

By increasing muscular strength, we increase flexibility and endurance. For example, you'll find that the first time you ride your bike from home to downtown, your legs may feel sore. Do that same ride ten times, and your legs will no longer ache. That's what's meant by building endurance. Of course, you won't be as out of breath, either, which is another sign of endurance.

Hand weights or resistance exercises help increase lean body mass—body tissue that is not fat. (See Item 16.) As your muscles become bigger, your body fat decreases. Because muscle is heavier than fat many people find their weight does not drop when they begin to exercise.

Sugar and Muscle

When you think "muscle," think "sugar." Every time you work any muscle in your body, either independent of an aerobic activity or during one, your muscles use up glucose from your bloodstream as fuel. People with high blood sugar prior to muscle toning will find that their blood sugar levels are lower after the muscles have been worked.

On the downside, if you have normal blood sugar levels prior to working a muscle, you may find that your blood sugar goes too low after you exercise unless you eat something. This should be a carbohydrate. In fact, your muscles prefer to use carbohydrates rather than fat as fuel. When your muscles use up all the sugar in your blood, your liver will convert glycogen (excess glucose it stores up for these kinds of emergencies) back into glucose and release it into your bloodstream for your muscles to use.

To avoid this scenario, eat before and after exercising if your blood sugar level is normal. How much you eat prior to exercising largely depends on what you're doing and how long you're going to be doing it. The general rule is to follow your meal plan, eating smaller, more frequent meals throughout the day to keep your blood sugar levels consistent.

Athletes without diabetes generally consume large quantities of carbohydrates before an intense workout. In fact, it's a known strategy in the athletic world to eat 40 to 65 grams of carbohydrate per hour to maintain blood glucose levels to the point where performance is improved. It's also been shown that ingesting glucose, sucrose, maltodextrins, or high-fructose corn syrup during exercise can increase endurance. After a training session, athletes typically consume more carbohydrates to replenish their energy and carry on throughout the day.

Athletes who have Type 1 diabetes do exactly the same thing, except they must be more careful about timing their food intake with insulin to avoid either low or high blood sugar.

If your blood sugar is low, don't exercise at all—this may be life threatening. Do not resume exercise until you get your blood sugar levels under control.

Exercises That Can Be Hazardous

Activities such as wrestling or weightlifting are usually short but very intense. As a result, unless you fuel up ahead of time, they will force your body to use glycogen, the stored glucose your liver keeps handy. When you have diabetes, it's not a great idea to force your liver to give up that glycogen. This can actually increase your blood pressure and put you at risk for other health problems, including hypoglycemia. To avoid this, you'll need to eat some carbohydrates prior to these activities, which will provide enough fuel to the muscles.

A Word About Leg Cramps

When your blood sugar is unstable, concentrations of sodium, potassium, and calcium can also "swing," which can cause leg cramps. Some things that aggravate leg cramps include:

- Diuretics, which can cause you to lose muscle potassium.
- Too much or too little intake of calcium.
- Sitting too long.

- Wearing high boots or knee socks.

- Varicose veins or pregnancy.

Be mindful of the factors above if you suffer from leg cramps. Experts recommend that increasing your potassium intake and stretching your leg muscles before going to bed can help to alleviate cramping.

14. More Ways to Increase Oxygen Flow

This will come as welcome news to people who have limited movement due to joint problems, arthritis, or other health complications ranging from stroke to kidney disease: You can increase the flow of oxygen into your bloodstream without exercising your heart muscle by learning how to breathe deeply through your diaphragm. There are many yogalike programs and videos available that can teach you this technique, which does not require you to jump around. The benefit is that you improve the oxygen flow into your bloodstream, which is better than doing nothing at all to improve your health and has many health benefits, according to a myriad of wellness practitioners.

15. Start Active Living Instead of Aerobic Living

The phrase *aerobic activity* means that the activity causes your heart to pump harder and faster and causes you to breathe faster, which increases oxygen flow. Activities such as cross-country skiing, walking, hiking, and biking are all aerobic.

But you know what? Exercise practitioners hate the terms *aerobic activity* and *aerobics program* because these are not things people do in their daily lives. Health promoters are replacing these terms with the phrase active living—because that's what becoming active is all about. There are many ways you can adopt an active lifestyle. Here are some suggestions:

- If you drive everywhere, pick the parking space furthest from your destination so you can work some daily walking into your life.

- If you take public transit everywhere, get off one or two stops early so you can walk the rest of the way to your destination.

- Choose stairs over escalators or elevators.

- Park at one side of the mall and then walk to the other.

- Take a stroll after dinner around your neighborhood.

- Volunteer to walk the dog.

- On weekends, go to the zoo or get out to flea markets, garage sales, and so on.

16. For Variety, Try Weight-Bearing Activities

You're not just exercising to work your heart muscle and increase oxygen flow, but to make your entire body stronger and more efficient. The side benefit to this is that you can prevent a whole host of health problems, including heart disease, a complication of diabetes. As mentioned earlier, "If you want a strong house, you need a strong frame." When you increase the load on your bones, your bones increase in mass; similarly, when you decrease the load on your bones, they decrease in mass. And the denser your bones, the harder they are to break. That's why exercises that build bone mass are important—and you use up calories to boot! By increasing muscular strength through these activities, we also increase flexibility (to help combat falls) and endurance.

As discussed above, hand weights or resistance exercises help increase lean body mass—body tissue that is not fat. Leg lifts and arm lifts with weights increase balance and bone strength and help maintain flexibility. Begin with 1-pound weights and increase slowly to 4 to 5 pounds.

Other forms of resistance exercise involve moving objects or your own body weight to create resistance, such as using equipment at a gym or fitness center or even common household objects such as water jugs or canned goods. Wearing Velcro weights on your wrists and ankles and just moving around as you normally would is also a good way to increase resistance.

As your muscles become bigger and your bones become denser, your body fat will decrease. Weight-bearing exercises should be done four times a week for thirty minutes per session.

Enjoyable Activities That May Help Build Bone Mass

Choose one activity from this list that is a pleasurable sport. If you enjoy your activity, you'll do it more often:

- Walking.
- Running.

- Jogging.
- Bicycling.
- Hiking.
- Tai chi.
- Cross-country skiing.
- Gardening.
- Weight lifting.
- Snowshoeing.
- Stair climbing.
- Tennis.
- Bowling.
- Rowing.
- Dancing.
- Water workouts.
- Badminton.
- Basketball.
- Volleyball.
- Soccer.

17. Know When to Consult a Fitness Practitioner

Many people may find it difficult to just dive into a brand-new fitness routine, particularly if they have diabetes or are taking medications that can affect their hearts. Intense exercise in these cases can be dangerous. If you're just beginning to incorporate exercise into your lifestyle after many years of being sedentary, a good route is to consult with a fitness practitioner, just as you would a nutritionist. Fitness practitioners can be found through your family doctor or through reputable fitness institutions. A fitness practitioner will plan an exercise regimen that is suited to your current physique and shape and will slowly increase your activity over time, as you build stamina. Working with a fitness practitioner also allows you to discuss your health conditions and any medications you're taking so your activities can complement, rather than aggravate, your health conditions.

18. Start Slow

More than 50 percent of all people with diabetes exercise less than once a week, and 56 percent of all diabetes-related deaths are due to heart attacks. This is terrible news, considering how beneficial and life extending exercise can be. Reports from the United States show that one out of three American adults is overweight, a sign of growing inactivity. Some people are so put off by the health club scene that they become even more sedentary. This is similar to diet failure, in which you become so demoralized after cheating that you binge even more.

What's the definition of sedentary? Not moving! If you have a desk job or spend most of your time at a computer, in your car, or watching television (even if it is PBS or CNN), you are a sedentary person. If you do roughly twenty minutes of exercise less than once a week, you're relatively sedentary. You need to incorporate some sort of movement into your daily schedule in order to be considered active. That movement can be anything: aerobic exercise, brisk walks around the block, or walking your dog. If you lead a sedentary lifestyle and are obese, you are at significant risk of developing Type 2 diabetes in your forties, if you are genetically predisposed. For women who are not obese, the risk is certainly lower, but they are then predisposed to a number of other problems. If you've been sedentary most of your life, there's nothing wrong with starting off with simple, even leisurely activities such as gardening, feeding the birds in a park, or a few simple stretches. Any step you take toward being more active is a crucial and important step.

Experts also recommend that you find a friend, neighbor, or relative to "get physical" with you. When your exercise plans include someone else, you'll be less apt to cancel them or make excuses for not getting out there.

Things to Do Before Moving Day

Choose an activity that's right for you. Whether it's walking, chopping wood, jumping rope, or folk dancing—pick something you enjoy. You don't have to do the same thing each time, either. Vary your routine to avoid monotony; just make sure that whatever activity you choose is continuous for the duration. Walking for two minutes, then stopping for three isn't continuous. It's also important to choose an activity that doesn't aggravate a preexisting problem, such as eye difficulties. Lowering your head in a certain way (as in touching your toes) or straining your upper body can increase blood pressure and/or aggravate eye troubles. If foot problems are a concern, an activity that doesn't involve walking, such as canoeing, is better—and so on.

- Choose the frequency. Decide how often you're going to do this activity. (Two, three, or four times a week? Or once a day?) Try not to let two days pass without doing something. Also, pick a duration. If you're elderly or ill, even a few minutes is a good start. If you're sedentary but otherwise healthy, aim for twenty to thirty minutes.

- Choose the intensity level that's right for you. If you're using an exercise machine of some kind, just set the dial. If you're walking, intensity is determined by how fast you walk, or how many hills you climb. In other words, how fast do you want your heart to beat?

- Coordinate activity with your meal plan. Once you decide what kind of exercise you'll be doing and for how long, see your dietitian about working your exercise into your current meal plan. You may need a small snack before and after exercise if you're planning to be active for longer than thirty minutes. If you are overweight, you do not need to consume extra calories before exercising unless your blood sugar level is low.

- Tell your doctor what you're doing. Your doctor may want to monitor your blood sugar more closely (or want you to do so), or adjust your medication. Don't do anything without consulting your doctor first.

19. Choose One Sport from This Table

TABLE 19.1 Suggested Activities

More intense	Less intense
Skiing	Golf
Running	Bowling
Jogging	Badminton
Stair stepping or Stair climbing	Croquet
Trampolining	Sailing
Jumping rope	Swimming
Fitness walking	Strolling
Race walking	Stretching
Aerobic classes	
Roller skating	
Ice skating	
Biking	
Weight-lifting exercises	
Tennis	
Swimming	

20. Try Some of These Variations on Jogging

- After warming up with a fifteen-minute walk, simply walk quickly with maximum exertion for two minutes, then slow down for one minute. Keep your heart rate up on the downhill portion of a walk or hike by adding lunges or squats.

- Vary the way you walk for coordination and balance. Try lifting the knees as high as you can, as if marching. Alternate with a shuffle, letting the tips of your fingers touch the ground as you walk. Do a sideways crab walk. To strengthen the rarely used muscles of the ankles and feet, walk first on the outsides, then on the insides of your feet. Or practice walking backwards.

- Use a curb for a step workout. Or climb stairs two at a time.

Water Workouts

- Start by walking in water that's relatively shallow (waist or chest deep). Your breathing and heartbeat will determine how hard you are working. Since you'll be moving fairly slowly, pay attention to your body.

- For all-over leg toning, take fifty steps forward, fifty steps sideways in crablike fashion, fifty steps backward, and then fifty steps to the other side.

- To tone your arms, submerge yourself from the neck down, bringing the arms in and out as if clapping. The water will provide natural resistance.

- Deep-water workouts are the most difficult, because every move you make is met with resistance. Wear a flotation vest and run without touching the bottom for optimum exertion and little or no impact.

- You may also want to try buoyant ankle cuffs and Styrofoam dumbbells or kickboards for full-body conditioning in the water.

- Deep relaxation and yoga breathing, such as alternate nostril breathing, calms the sympathetic nervous system, thus relaxing the small arteries, and permanently lowers blood pressure.

PART THREE

Meal Planning

21. Understand the Goal of Meal Plans

Meal plans recommended by registered dietitians are tailored to your individual goals and medication regimen. Men and women usually require different quantities of food. The goal is to keep the supply of glucose consistent by spacing out your meals, snacks, and activity levels accordingly. Losing weight will allow your body to use insulin more effectively, but not all people with Type 2 diabetes need to lose weight. If you're on insulin, meals need to be timed to match your insulin's peak. A dietitian can help by prescribing an individualized meal plan that addresses your specific needs (weight control, shift work, travel, and so on).

A good meal plan will ensure that you are getting enough nutrients to meet your energy needs and that your food is spread out over the course of the day. For example, if your meal plan allows for three meals with one to two snacks, meals should be spaced four to six hours apart so your body isn't overwhelmed. If you are obese, snacks will likely be discouraged because they can cause you to oversecrete insulin and increase your appetite. A meal plan should also help you to eat consistently rather than bingeing one day and starving the next.

A good meal plan will also ensure that you're getting the vitamins and minerals you need without taking vitamin and mineral supplements.

Golden Rules of Diabetes Meal Plans

- Eat three meals a day at fairly regular times (spaced four to six hours apart).
- Ask your dietitian to help you plan your snacks.
- Try to eat a variety of foods each day from all food groups.
- Learn how to gauge serving sizes, volume of bowls and glasses, and so on.
- Ask your dietitian or diabetes educator about how to adjust your diet if you're traveling (this depends on whether you take medication, where you're going, what foods will be available, and so on).
- Draw up a "sick days plan" with your dietitian. This will depend on what your regular meal plan includes.
- Ask about any meal supplements, such as breakfast bars, sports bars, or meal replacement drinks. How will these figure into your meal plan?
- Choose low-fat foods often.

22. Understand Sugars

Sugars are found naturally in many foods you eat. The simplest form of sugar is glucose, which is what blood sugar, also called blood glucose, is—your basic body fuel. You can buy pure glucose at any drugstore in the form of dextrose tablets. Dextrose is edible glucose. For example, when people are fed sugar water intravenously, dextrose is the sugar in that water. When you see dextrose on a candy-bar label, it means that the candy-bar manufacturer used edible glucose in the recipe.

Glucose is the baseline ingredient of all naturally occurring sugars, which include:

- Sucrose: table or white sugar, naturally found in sugar cane and sugar beets.

- Fructose: the natural sugar in fruits and vegetables.

- Lactose: the natural sugar in all milk products.

- Maltose: the natural sugar in grains (flours and cereals).

When you ingest a natural sugar of any kind, you're actually ingesting one part glucose and one or two parts of another naturally occurring sugar. For example, sucrose is biochemically constructed from one part glucose and one part fructose. So, from glucose it came, and unto glucose it shall return—once it hits your digestive system. The same is true for all naturally occurring sugars, with the exception of lactose. As it happens, lactose breaks down into glucose and an "odd duck" simple sugar, galactose (which I used to think was something in our solar system until I became a health writer). Just think of lactose as the Milky Way and you'll probably remember.

Simple sugars can get pretty complicated when you discuss their molecular structures. For example, simple sugars can be classified as monosaccharides (single sugars) or dissaccharides (double sugars). But unless you're writing a chemistry exam on sugars, you don't need to know this confusing stuff: You just need to know that all naturally occurring sugars wind up as glucose once you eat them; glucose is carried to your cells through the bloodstream and is used as body fuel or energy.

How long does it take for one of the above sugars to return to glucose? It greatly depends on the amount of fiber in your food, how much protein you've eaten, and how much fat accompanies the sugar in your meal. If you have enough energy or fuel, once that sugar becomes glucose, it can be stored as fat. And that's how—and why—sugar can make you fat.

Factory-Added Sugars

What you have to watch out for is added sugar; these are sugars that manufacturers add to foods during processing or packaging. Foods containing fruit juice concentrates, invert sugar, regular corn syrup, honey, molasses, hydrolyzed lactose syrup, or high-fructose corn syrup (made out of highly concentrated fructose through the hydrolysis of starch) all have added sugars. Many people don't realize, however, that pure, unsweetened fruit juice is still a potent source of sugar, even when it contains no added sugar. Extra lactose (naturally occurring sugar in milk products), dextrose (edible glucose), and maltose (naturally occurring sugar in grains) are also in many of your foods. In other words, the products may have naturally occurring sugars anyway, and then more sugar is thrown in to enhance consistency, taste, and so on. The best way to know how much sugar is in a product is to look on the nutritional label under total carbohydrates.

Why Is Sugar Added?

Sugar is added to food because it can change the consistency of foods and, in some instances, act as a preservative, as in jams and jellies. Sugars increase the boiling point or reduce the freezing point in foods; they add bulk and density and make baked goods do wonderful things, including helping yeast to ferment. Sugar can also add moisture to dry foods, making them crisp, or balance acidic tastes found in foods such as tomato sauce or salad dressing. Both invert sugar and corn syrup are used to prevent sucrose from crystallizing in candy.

Since the 1950s, a popular natural sugar in North America has been fructose, which has replaced sucrose in many food products in the form of high-fructose syrup (HFS), made from corn. HFS was developed in response to high sucrose prices and is very cheap to make. In other parts of the world, the equivalent of high-fructose syrup is made from whatever starches are local, such as rice, tapioca, wheat, or cassava. According to the International Food Information Council in Washington, D.C., the average North American consumes about 37 grams of fructose daily.

23. Understand Fat

Fat is technically known as fatty acids, which are crucial nutrients for our cells. We cannot live without fatty acids, or fat. If you looked at each fat molecule carefully, you'd find three different kinds of fatty acids in it: saturated (solid), monounsaturated (less solid, with the exception of olive and peanut oils), and polyunsaturated (liquid) fatty acids. The term *unsaturated fat* refers to either monounsaturated or polyunsaturated fats.

These three fatty acids combine with glycerol to make what's chemically known as triglycerides. Each fat molecule is a link in a chain made up of glycerol, carbon atoms, and hydrogen atoms. The more hydrogen atoms that are on that chain, the more saturated or solid the fat. The liver breaks down fat molecules by secreting bile (stored in the gall-bladder)—its sole function. The liver also makes cholesterol. Too much saturated fat may cause your liver to overproduce cholesterol, while the triglycerides in your bloodstream will rise, perpetuating the problem.

Fat is therefore a good thing—in moderation. But like all good things, most of us want too much of it. Excess dietary fat is by far the most damaging element in the Western diet. A gram of fat contains twice the calories as the same amount of protein or carbohydrate. Decreasing the fat in your diet and replacing it with more grain products, vegetables, and fruit is the best way to lower your risk of colon cancer and cardiovascular diseases. Fat in the diet comes from meats, dairy products, and vegetable oils. Other sources of fat include coconuts (60 percent fat), peanuts (78 percent fat), and avocados (82 percent fat). There are different kinds of fatty acids in these sources of fats: saturated, monounsaturated, and polyunsaturated. And then there is a fourth kind of fat in our diets: trans-fatty acids, the factory-made fat found in margarine.

To cut through all this fat jargon, you can boil down fat into two categories: harmful fats and helpful fats (which the popular press often defines as good fats and bad fats).

Harmful Fats

The following are harmful fats because they can increase your risk of cardiovascular problems, as well as many cancers, including colon and breast cancers. These fats are fine in moderation, but harmful in excess:

- Saturated fats. These are solid at room temperature and stimulate cholesterol production in your body. In fact, the way that saturated fat looks before ingesting it is the way it will look when it lines your arteries. Foods high in saturated fat include processed meat, fatty meat, lard, butter, margarine, solid vegetable shortening, chocolate, and tropical oils (coconut oil is more than 90 percent saturated). Saturated fat should be consumed only in very small amounts.

- Trans-fatty acids. These are factory-made fats that behave just like saturated fat in your body. (See next page for details.)

Helpful Fats

These fats are beneficial to your health and actually protect against certain health problems, such as cardiovascular disease. You are encouraged to use these fats more, rather than less frequently in your diet. In fact, nutritionists suggest that you substitute these for harmful fats.

- Unsaturated fat. This is partially solid or liquid at room temperature. The more liquid the fat, the more polyunsaturated it is, which, in fact, lowers your cholesterol levels. This group of fats includes monounsaturated fats and polyunsaturated fats. Sources of unsaturated fats include vegetable oils (canola, saf-flower, sunflower, corn, olive) and seeds and nuts. Un-saturated fats come from plants, with the exception of tropical oils, such as coconut.

- Fish fats (omega-3 oils). The fats naturally present in fish that swim in cold waters, known as omega-3 fatty acids or fish oils, are all polyunsaturated. Again, poly-unsaturated fats are good for you: They lower choles-terol levels, are crucial for brain tissue, and protect against heart disease. Look for cold-water fish, such as mackerel, albacore tuna, salmon, and sardines.

Avoid Factory-Made Fats

An assortment of factory-made fats have been introduced into our diets, courtesy of food producers who are trying to give us the taste of fat without all the problems associated with saturated fats. Unfortunately, man-made fats offer their own bag of horrors. When a fat is made in a factory, it becomes a trans-fatty acid, a harmful fat that not only raises the level of bad cholesterol (LDL, short for low-density lipoproteins) in your bloodstream, but lowers the amount of good cholesterol (HDL, short for high-density lipoproteins) that's already there.

How, exactly, does a trans-fatty acid come into being? Trans-fatty acids are what you get when you make a liquid oil, such as corn oil, into a more solid or spreadable sub-stance, such as margarine. Trans-fatty acids, you might say, are the "road to hell, paved with good intentions." Someone, way back when, thought that if you could take the good fat—unsaturated fat—and solidify it so it could double as butter or lard, you could eat the same things without missing the spreadable, but saturated fat. That sounds like a great idea. Unfortunately, to make an unsaturated liquid fat more solid, you have to add hydrogen to its molecules, a process called hydrogenation. That ever-popular chocolate bar ingredient, hydrogenated palm oil, is a classic example of a trans-fatty acid. Hydrogenation also prolongs the shelf life of fats, such as polyunsaturated fats, which can oxidize when exposed to air, causing rancid odors or flavors. Deep-frying oils used in the restaurant trade are generally hydrogenated.

What's Wrong with Trans-Fatty Acid?

Trans-fatty acid is sold as a polyunsaturated or monounsaturated fat with a line of advertising copy such as, "Made from polyunsaturated vegetable oil." The problem is your body treats it as a saturated fat. So trans-fatty acids are really saturated fats in disguise. The advertiser may, in fact, say that the product contains no saturated fat or is healthier than the comparable animal or tropical oil product with saturated fat. So be careful out there: *read your labels*. The magic word you're looking for is hydrogenated. If the product lists a variety of unsaturated fats (monounsaturated X oil, polyunsaturated Y oil, and so on), keep reading. If the word *hydrogenated* appears, count that product as a saturated fat; your body will!

Margarine Versus Butter

There's an old tongue twister: "Betty Botter bought some butter that made the batter bitter; so Betty Botter bought more butter that made the batter better." Are we making our batters bitter or better with margarine? It depends.

Since the news of trans-fatty acids broke in the late 1980s, margarine manufacturers began to offer some less "bitter" margarines; some contain no hydrogenated oils, while others have much smaller amounts. Margarines with less than 60 to 80 percent oil (9 to 11 grams of fat) contain 1 to 3 grams of trans-fatty acids per serving, compared to butter, which is 53 percent saturated fat. You might say it's a choice between a bad fat and a worse fat.

It's also possible for a liquid vegetable oil to retain a high concentration of unsaturated fat when it's been partially hydrogenated. In this case, your body will metabolize this as some saturated fat and some unsaturated fat.

Fake Fat

We have artificial sweeteners; why not artificial fat? This question has led to the creation of an emerging yet highly suspicious ingredient: the fat substitute, designed to replace real fat and hence reduce calories without compromising taste. This is accomplished by creating a fake fat that the body cannot absorb.

One of the first fat substitutes was Simplesse, an all-natural fat substitute made from milk and egg-white protein, which was developed by the NutraSweet Company. Simplesse apparently adds one to two calories per gram instead of the usual nine calories per gram from fat. Other fat substitutes simply take protein and carbohydrates and modify them in some way to simulate the textures of fat (creamy, smooth, and so on). All these fat substitutes help to create some low-fat products.

The calorie-free fat substitute presently being promoted is called Olestra, developed by Procter & Gamble. It's currently being test-marketed in the United States in a variety of savory snacks such as potato chips and crackers. Olestra is a potentially dangerous ingredient that most experts feel can do more harm than good. Canada has not yet approved it.

Olestra is made from a combination of vegetable oils and sugar. It tastes just like the real thing, but the biochemical structure is a molecule too big for your liver to break down. So, Olestra just gets passed into the large intestine and is excreted. Olestra is more than an "empty" molecule, however. According to the FDA Commissioner of Food and Drugs, Olestra may cause diarrhea and cramps and may deplete your body of vital nutrients, including vitamins A, D, E, and K (necessary for blood to clot). Indeed, all studies conducted by Procter & Gamble have shown this potential. If the FDA approves Olestra for use as a cooking-oil substitute, you'll see it in every imaginable high-fat product. Another danger with Olestra was raised by nutritionists in a critique published in 1996 (the year Olestra was approved for test markets), in an issue of the University of California at Berkeley *Wellness Letter*. Instead of encouraging people to choose nutritious foods, such as fruits, grains, and vegetables over high-fat foods, products such as these encourage a high-fake-fat diet that's still too low in fiber and other essential nutrients. The no-fat icing on the cake is that these people could potentially wind up with a vitamin deficiency to boot. Products such as Olestra should make you nervous.

24. Cut Down on Carbs

Fat is not the only thing that can make you fat; what about carbohydrates? You see, a diet high in carbohydrates can also make you fat. That's because carbohydrates—starchy stuff, such as rice, pasta, breads, and potatoes—can be stored as fat when eaten in excess.

Carbohydrates can be simple or complex. Simple carbohydrates are found in any food that has natural sugar (honey, fruits, juices, vegetables, and milk) and anything that contains table sugar.

Complex carbohydrates are more sophisticated foods that are made up of larger molecules, such as grain foods, starches, and foods high in fiber.

Normally, all carbs convert into glucose when you eat them. Glucose is the technical term for simplest sugar. All your energy comes from glucose in your blood—also known as blood glucose or blood sugar—your body fuel. When your blood sugar is used up, you feel weak and tired—and hungry. But what happens when you eat more carbohydrates than your body can use? Your body will store those extra carbs as fat. We also know that the rate at which glucose is absorbed by your body from carbohydrates is affected by other parts of your meal, such as its protein, fiber, and fat. If you're eating only carbohydrates and no protein or fat, for example, they will convert into glucose more quickly—to the point where you may feel mood swings as your blood sugar rises and dips.

Nutrition experts advise that each day you should consume roughly 50 to 55 percent carbohydrates, 15 to 20 percent protein, and less than 30 percent fat for a healthy diet.

25. Learn the Exchange System

The first thing you need to learn before you shop for food is the exchange system, developed by the American Diabetes Association, which tells you how various foods can be incorporated into your meal plan. (This is different than the Food Choice Value System symbols used by the Canadian Diabetes Association, in case you're shopping in Canada.) There are seven exchange list categories:

I. **Starches list.** Includes cereals, grains, pasta, breads, crackers, snacks, and starchy vegetables, such as legumes (peas and beans), potatoes, corn, and squash.

II. **Meat and meat substitutes list.** Includes poultry, fish, shellfish, game, beef, pork, lamb, cheese, tofu, tempeh, low-fat cheeses, egg whites, and soy milk.

III. **Fruit list.** Includes fresh fruit, frozen fruit, canned fruit, dried fruit, and juice. (Remember, fruit is any produce that grows on trees, vines, or plants, including tomatoes!)

IV. **Dairy list.** Includes most milk products.

V. **Vegetable list.** Includes most vegetables from A (for artichoke) to Z (for zucchini), but does not include starchy vegetables. (See Starches list.)

VI. **Fats list.** Includes monounsaturated fats, polyunsaturated fats, and saturated fats, based on the main type of fat any food contains.

VII. **Other carbohydrates.** Includes cakes, pies, puddings, granola bars, gelatin, and so on. This list includes any food that contains more fats and sugars than vitamins and minerals.

Your dietitian or diabetes educator will work with you to create an individual meal plan built around the above exchange lists. One person, for example, may eat for breakfast two items from List I, three items from List II, and two items from List VI; another person may require a completely different plan. I cannot tell you, in this book, how many items from the above lists you can have; I can only explain how the foods are categorized.

Your dietitian or diabetes educator should also teach you how to incorporate carbohydrate counting into meal planning, which can be done by learning to read labels properly, setting goals for a certain number of carbohydrates per day, and keeping accurate records of your blood sugar levels. (See Part One.)

The best advice regarding exchange lists is to purchase the American Diabetes Association's *Exchange Lists for Meal Planning* (the exchange list bible). It can be ordered directly from the American Diabetes Association by calling 1-800-232-6733.

26. Understand Sweeteners

We gravitate toward sweet flavors because we start out with the slightly sweet taste of breast milk. A product can be sweet without containing a drop of sugar, thanks to the invention of artificial sugars and sweeteners. Artificial sweeteners will not affect your blood sugar levels because they do not contain sugar; they may contain a tiny number of calories, however. It depends on whether that sweetener is classified as nutritive or nonnutritive.

Nutritive sweeteners have calories or contain natural sugar. White or brown table sugar, molasses, honey, and syrup are all considered nutritive sweeteners. Sugar alcohols (see page 57) are also nutritive sweeteners because they are made from fruits or produced commercially from dextrose. Sorbitol, mannitol, xylitol, and maltitol are all sugar alcohols. Sugar alcohols contain only four calories per gram, like ordinary sugar, and will affect your blood sugar levels like ordinary sugar. It all depends on how much is consumed and the degree of absorption from your digestive tract.

Nonnutritive sweeteners are sugar substitutes or artificial sweeteners; they do not have any calories and will not affect your blood sugar levels. Examples of nonnutritive sweeteners are saccharin, cyclamate, aspartame, sucralose, and acesulflame potassium.

The Sweetener Wars

The oldest nonnutritive sweetener is saccharin, which is what you get when you purchase Sweet 'n' Low or Hermesetas. Saccharin is 300 times sweeter than sucrose (table sugar) but has a metallic aftertaste. At one point in the 1970s, saccharin was also thought to cause cancer, but this was never proven.

In the 1980s, aspartame was invented, which is sold as NutraSweet. It is considered a nutritive sweetener because it is derived from natural sources (two amino acids, aspartic acid and phenylalanine), which means that aspartame is digested and metabolized the same as any other protein food. For every gram of aspartame, there are four calories. But since aspartame is 200 times sweeter than sugar, you don't need very much of it to achieve the desired sweetness.

In at least ninety countries, aspartame is found in more than one hundred fifty product categories, including breakfast cereals, beverages, desserts, candy, gum, syrups, salad dressings, and various snack foods. Here's where it gets confusing: Aspartame is also available as a tabletop sweetener under the brand name Equal and, most recently, Prosweet. An interesting point about aspartame is that it's not recommended for baking or any other recipe in which heat is required; the two amino acids in it separate when heated and the product loses its sweetness. That's not to say it's harmful if heated, but your recipe won't turn out.

For the moment, aspartame is considered safe for everybody, including people with diabetes, pregnant women, and children. The only people who are cautioned against consuming it are those with a rare hereditary disease known as phenylketonuria (PKU) because aspartame contains phenylalanine, which people with PKU cannot tolerate.

Another common tabletop sweetener is sucralose, sold as Splenda. Splenda is a white crystalline powder, actually made from sugar itself. It's 600 times sweeter than table sugar but is not broken down in your digestive system, so it has no calories at all. Splenda can also be used in hot or cold foods and is found in hot and cold beverages, frozen foods, baked goods, and other packaged foods.

In the United States, you can still purchase cyclamate, a nonnutritive sweetener sold under the brand name Sucaryl or Sugar Twin. Cyclamate is also the sweetener used in many weight control products and is thirty times sweeter than table sugar, with no aftertaste. Cyclamate is fine for hot or cold foods.

Sugar Alcohols

Not to be confused with alcoholic beverages, sugar alcohols are nutritive sweeteners, like regular sugar. These are found naturally in fruits or manufactured from carbohydrates. Sorbitol, mannitol, xylitol, maltitol, maltitol syrup, lactitol, isomalt, and hydrogenated starch hydrolysates are all sugar alcohols. In your body, these sugars are absorbed in the lower part of the digestive tract and will cause gastrointestinal symptoms if you use too much. Because sugar alcohols are absorbed slowly, they were once touted as ideal for people with diabetes. But since they are carbohydrates, they still increase your blood sugar—just like regular sugar. Now that artificial sweeteners are on the market in abundance, the only real advantage of sugar alcohols is that they don't cause cavities. The bacteria in your mouth doesn't like sugar alcohols as much as real sugar.

According to the FDA, even foods that contain sugar alcohols can be labeled "sugar free." Sugar alcohol products can also be labeled "Does not promote tooth decay," which is often confused with low calorie.

27. Plan for Alcohol

The one thing missing from the exchange lists is alcohol. As a food choice, alcohol is almost as fattening as an item from the Fats list, delivering about 7 calories per gram or 150 calories per drink. Many people with diabetes think they have to avoid alcohol completely because it converts into glucose. This is not so; alcohol alone doesn't increase blood sugar since alcohol cannot be turned into glucose. It's the sugar in an alcoholic beverage that can affect blood sugar level. The problem with alcohol is that it's so darned fattening, it's something people with Type 2 diabetes may need to avoid. That said, alcohol has been proven to raise your good cholesterol (HDL). This fact was discovered in the late 1980s when researchers probed why France, with all its rich food, had such low rates of heart disease. It was the wine; red wine, in particular, was shown to decrease the risk of cardiovascular disease. But any alcohol will do this, so it's okay to have this stuff, so long as you plan for it with your dietitian, discuss it with your doctor, and count it as an actual food choice.

It's crucial to note that alcohol can cause hypoglycemia (low blood sugar) if you're on oral hypoglycemic agents or insulin. Please discuss the effects of alcohol and hypoglycemia with your health care team.

Fine Wine

Dry wines generally mean no added sugar, but check with the wine producer if you're unsure. Dry wine is fine to ingest if you are diabetic. Wine is the result of natural sugar in fruits or fruit juices fermenting. Fermentation means that natural sugar is converted into alcohol. A glass of dry red or white wine has calories (discussed below) but no sugar. Unless sugar is added to the wine, there's no way that alcohol will change back into sugar, even in your digestive tract. The same thing goes for cognac, brandy, and dry sherry that contain no sugar.

On the other hand, a sweet wine usually contains about 3 grams of sugar per 3.5-ounce portion. Dessert wines or ice wines are really sweet; they contain about 15 percent sugar, or 10 grams of sugar for a 2-ounce serving. Sweet liqueurs are 35 percent sugar. A glass of dry wine with your meal adds about one hundred calories, or the equivalent calories of fat or oil. Half soda water and half wine (a spritzer) contains half the calories. When you cook with wine, the alcohol evaporates, leaving only the flavor. If your wine has no sugar, it counts as an item from the Fats list. If it has sugar, it counts as an item from both the Other Carbohydrates list as well as an item from the Fats list.

At the Pub

If you're a beer drinker, you're basically having some corn, barley, and a couple of teaspoons of malt sugar (maltose) when you have a bottle of beer. The corn and barley ferment into mostly alcohol and some maltose. Calorie-wise, that's about one hundred fifty calories per bottle plus 3 teaspoons of malt sugar. Beer can be defined as an item from the Other Carbohydrates list, plus an item from the Fats list.

A light beer has fewer calories but contains at least one hundred calories per bottle. Dealcoholized beer still has sugar and counts as an item from the Fruit list.

The Hard Stuff

The stiffer the drink, the fatter it gets. Hard liquors, such as scotch, rye, gin, and rum, are made out of cereal grains; vodka, the Russian staple, is made out of potatoes. In this case, the grains ferment into alcohol. Hard liquor averages about 40 percent alcohol, but has no sugar. Nevertheless, you're looking at about one hundred calories per small shot glass, so long as you don't add fruit juice, tomato or Clamato juice, or sugary soft drinks. As bizarre as it sounds, a Bloody Mary or Bloody Caesar is actually an item from the Starches list—potatoes—and Fruit list—tomatoes!

The Glycogen Factor

Glycogen is the stored sugar your liver keeps handy for emergencies. If your blood sugar needs a boost, the liver will tap into its glycogen stores and convert it into glucose. Alcohol in the liver blocks this conversion process. So, if you've been exercising, and then go out with friends for a few drinks, unless you've eaten something after your exercise, you may need that glycogen. If you drink to the point of feeling tipsy, that glycogen can be cut off by the alcohol, causing hypoglycemia. What complicates matters even more is that your hypoglycemia symptoms can mimic drunkenness. This glycogen problem can affect both people with Type 1 or Type 2 diabetes because it can result when either insulin or oral hypoglycemic agents are used.

28. Don't Drink and Starve

If you're going to drink, *eat*! Always have food with alcohol. Food delays absorption of alcohol into the bloodstream, providing you with carbohydrates and thereby preventing hypoglycemia.

Experts also recommend the following:

• Avoid alcohol when your blood sugar is high.

- Remember that two drinks a day is fine for someone with a healthy liver, but less is recommended for liver health.

- Choose dry wines or alcoholic beverages with no sugar. (Or rum and diet cola versus rum and regular cola.)

- Remember that juice has sugar; even tomato and Clamato juice.

- Never substitute alcohol for food if you're taking insulin or pills.

- Don't be afraid to ask your dietitian about how to count your favorite wine or cocktail as a food choice. Again, as long as it's planned for, it's fine.

- Talk to your doctor about how to safely balance alcohol and insulin, and alcohol and oral hypoglycemic agents.

29. Understand How Your Food Breaks Down

A good way to help you gauge how quickly your food converts to glucose is to use the glycemic index (see Exhibit 29.1). The glycemic index (GI) shows the rise in blood sugar from various carbohydrates. Therefore, planning your diet using the GI can help you control your blood sugar by using more foods with a low GI and fewer foods with a high GI. Nutritionists report that this is useful as a tool in meal planning.

You can also use Table 29.1 as a guideline for how fast your food breaks down, so you can plan for your meals better according to ADA guidelines.

EXHIBIT 29.1 The Glycemic Index at a Glance

This glycemic index, developed at the University of Toronto, measures the rate at which various foods convert to glucose, which is assigned a value of 100. Higher numbers indicate a more rapid absorption of glucose. This is not an exhaustive list and should be used as a sample only. This is not an index of food energy values or calories; some low GI foods are high in fat, while some high GI foods are low in fat. Keep in mind, too, that these values differ depending on what else you're eating with that food and how the food is prepared.

Sugars

Glucose = 100
Honey = 87
Table sugar = 59
Fructose = 20

Snacks

Mars bar = 68
Potato chips = 51
Sponge cake = 46
Fish sticks = 38
Tomato soup = 38
Sausages = 28
Peanuts = 13

Cereals

Cornflakes = 80
Shredded wheat = 67
Muesli = 66
All Bran = 51
Oatmeal = 49

Breads

Whole wheat = 72
White = 69
Buckwheat = 51

Fruits

Raisins = 64
Banana = 62
Orange juice = 46
Orange = 40
Apple = 39

Dairy Products

Ice cream = 36
Yogurt = 36
Milk = 34
Nonfat milk = 32

Root Vegetables

Parsnips = 97
Carrots = 92
Instant mashed potatoes = 80
New boiled potato = 70
Beets = 64
Yam = 51
Sweet potato = 48

Pasta and Rice

White rice = 72
Brown rice = 66
Spaghetti (white) = 50
Spaghetti (whole wheat) = 42

Legumes

Frozen peas = 51
Baked beans = 40
Chickpeas = 36
Lima beans = 36
Butter beans = 36
Black-eyed peas = 33
Green beans = 31
Kidney beans = 29
Lentils = 29
Dried soybeans = 15

TABLE 29.1 How Your Food Breaks Down

Complex Carbohydrates (digest slowly)	Defined by ADA
fruits	Fruit list
vegetables (corn, potatoes, and so on)	Vegetable list or Starches list
grains (breads, pastas, and cereals)	Starches list
legumes (dried beans, peas, and lentils)	Starches list

Simple Carbohydrates (digest quickly)	Defined by ADA
fruits/fruit juices	Fruit list
sugars (sucrose, fructose, and so on)	Fruit/Other Carbohydrates/Starches lists
honey	Fruit/Other Carbohydrates/Starches lists
corn syrup	Fruit/Other Carbohydrates/Starches lists
sorghum	Fruit/Other Carbohydrates/Starches lists
date sugar	Fruit/Other Carbohydrates/Starches lists
molasses	Fruit/Other Carbohydrates/Starches lists
lactose	Dairy list

Proteins (digest slowly)	Defined by ADA
lean meats	Meat and Meat Substitutes list
fatty meats	Meat and Meat Substitutes/Fats lists
poultry	Meat and Meat Substitutes list
fish	Meat and Meat Substitutes list
eggs	Meat and Meat Substitutes list
low-fat cheese	Meat and Meat Substitutes list
regular cheese	Dairy list or Fats list
legumes	Starches list
grains	Starches list

Fats (digest slowly)	Defined by ADA
high-fat dairy products (butter or cream)	Dairy list or Fats list
oils (canola/corn/olive/safflower/sunflower)	Fats list
lard	Fats list
avocados	Fats list or Vegetable list
olives	Fats list or Vegetable list
nuts	Fats list or Vegetable list
fatty meats	Fats/Meat and Meat Substitutes lists

continued on next page

TABLE 29.1 How Your Food Breaks Down continued

Fiber (doesn't digest; goes through you)	Defined by ADA
whole-grain breads	Starches list
cereals (for example, oatmeal)	Starches list
all fruits	Fruit list
legumes (beans and lentils)	Starches list
leafy greens	Vegetable list
cruciferous vegetables	Vegetable list

30. Know the Importance of Fiber in Blood Sugar Control

Soluble fiber helps delay glucose from being absorbed into your bloodstream, which not only improves blood sugar control but helps to control postmeal peaks in blood sugar, which stimulate the pancreas to produce more insulin. Fiber in the form of all colors of vegetables will also ensure that you're getting the right mix of nutrients. Experts suggest that you have a variety of colors of vegetables daily—for example, carrots, beets, and spinach. An easy way to remember what nutrients are in which vegetable is to remember that all green vegetables are for cellular repair; the darker the green, the more nutrients the vegetable contains. All red, orange, and purplish vegetables contain antioxidants (vitamins A, C, and E) that boost the immune system and fight off toxins. Studies suggest that vitamin C, for example, is crucial for people with Type 2 diabetes because it helps to prevent complications, as well as rid the body of sorbitol, which can increase blood sugar. Another study suggests that vitamin E helps to prevent heart disease in people with Type 2 diabetes by lowering levels of bad cholesterol (LDL), but this has not yet been conclusively proven. Other minerals, such as zinc and copper, are essential for wound healing. The recommendation is to eat all colors of vegetables in ample amounts to get your vitamins, minerals, and dietary fiber. This makes sense when you understand diabetes as a disease of starvation. In starvation, there are naturally lower levels of nutrients in your body that can only be replenished through excellent sources of food.

Soluble Versus Insoluble Fiber

Soluble and insoluble fiber do differ, but they are both equally good. Soluble fiber—somehow—lowers the bad cholesterol, or LDL, in your body. Experts aren't entirely sure how soluble fiber works its magic, but one popular theory is that it gets mixed into the bile the liver secretes and forms a type of gel that traps the building blocks of cholesterol, thus lowering LDL levels. It's akin to a spider web trapping smaller insects. Sources of soluble fiber include oats and oat bran, legumes (dried beans and peas), some seeds, carrots, oranges, bananas, and other fruits. Soybeans are also good sources of soluble fiber. Studies show that people with very high cholesterol have the most to gain by eating soybeans. Soybeans also contain a phytoestrogen (plant estrogen) that is believed to lower the risks of estrogen-related cancers (for example, breast cancer), as well as lower the incidence of estrogen-loss symptoms associated with menopause.

Whole-grain breads are also good sources of insoluble fiber (flax bread is particularly good because flaxseeds are a source of soluble fiber, too). The problem is understanding what is truly whole grain. For example, there is an assumption that if bread is dark or brown, it's more nutritious; this isn't so. In fact, many brown breads are simply enriched white breads dyed with molasses. (Enriched means that nutrients lost during processing have been replaced.) High-fiber pita breads and bagels are available, but you have to search for them.

PART FOUR

Diabetes Medications and Insulin

31. Know What Is Meant by Diabetes Medications

There are four kinds of medications that may be prescribed to you. It's crucial to note, however, that these medications can only be prescribed to people who still produce insulin. They have no effect on people with Type 1, or insulin-dependent diabetes. When diet and lifestyle changes make no impact on your blood sugar levels, you may be prescribed pills.

Before you fill your prescription for antidiabetes pills, you should know that between 40 and 50 percent of all people with Type 2 diabetes require insulin therapy after ten years. Continuing insulin resistance may cause you to stop responding to oral medications. Furthermore, these pills are meant to complement your meal plan, exercise routine, and glucose monitoring; they are not a substitute.

Bear in mind, too, that physicians who prescribe the medications discussed in this section, without also working with you to modify your diet and lifestyle, are not managing your diabetes properly. These medications should be prescribed only after you've been unsuccessful in managing your Type 2 diabetes through lifestyle modification and frequent blood sugar testing.

If you cannot get down to a healthy body weight, you are probably a good candidate for antidiabetes medication. In addition, anyone with Type 2 diabetes who cannot control his or her blood sugar levels despite lifestyle changes is also a good candidate for the drugs discussed below.

32. Understand Oral Hypoglycemic Agents (OHAs)

Sulphonylureas and biguanides are common oral hypoglycemic agents (OHAs). Sulphonylureas are pills that help your pancreas release more insulin; biguanides help your insulin work better. Initially, 75 percent of people with Type 2 diabetes will respond well to sulphonylureas, while biguanides will lower blood sugar in 80 percent of people with Type 2 diabetes. But about 15 percent of all people treated with OHAs fail to respond to them at all, while 3 to 5 percent will stop responding to them each year. So don't get too comfortable on these pills.

Sulphonylureas are generally the initial oral agent of choice for people who are not obese and/or have high blood sugar levels (or suffer from symptoms of high blood sugar). A biguanide is appropriate for people who are obese and have milder levels of high blood sugar. That's because biguanides do not result in weight gain, which is typically associated with sulphonylurea and insulin therapy.

Dosages for Sulphonylureas

There is no fixed dosage for sulphonylureas; it all depends on the brand prescribed. For example, it's perfectly common to take anything from 80 to 320 mg a day. If you are taking a dosage higher than the usual initial dose, you should divide your dose into two equal parts. Your pills should be taken before or with meals, and your doctor should start you on the lowest effective dose. If your blood sugar levels are high when you start your pills, it's a good idea to have a short trial period of about six to eight weeks to make sure the drug is working.

Dosages for Biguanides (Metformin)

The most common biguanide available goes by the trade name Metformin. In this case, the usual dose is 500 mg three or four times a day or 850 mg two or three times a day. Your dose should not exceed 2.5 g a day. If you're elderly, a lower dose will probably be prescribed.

When OHAs Should Not Be Used

If you've had Type 2 diabetes longer than ten years, this is not the time to start OHAs. And, of course, nobody with Type 1 or insulin-dependent diabetes (IDDM) should ever take OHAs; they will not work. OHAs should also never be taken under the following conditions:

- Alcoholism.
- Pregnancy.
- Kidney or liver failure (Metformin only).

Side Effects

Sixty percent of people taking OHAs continue to have high blood sugar levels two hours after meals. These pills can also cause increased appetite and weight gain. The main side effect with first-generation OHAs, however, is hypoglycemia (low blood sugar), which occurs in one in five people treated with OHAs. If you're over age sixty, hypoglycemia may occur more often, which is why it's dangerous for anyone over age seventy to take certain OHAs.

About one-third of all people taking OHAs experience gastrointestinal side effects (loss of appetite, nausea, abdominal discomfort, and, with Metformin, diarrhea). Adjusting dosages and taking pills with your meals or afterward often clear up these symptoms.

33. Ask About Acarbose (Alpha-Glucosidase Inhibitors)

Acarbose is a pill that delays the breakdown of sugar in your meal by delaying the conversion of starch and sucrose into glucose. This reduces high blood sugar levels after you eat. Acarbose is prescribed to people who cannot seem to get their after-meal (that is, postmeal or postprandial) blood sugar down to acceptable levels. A major benefit of acarbose is that it may reduce the risk of hypoglycemic episodes during the night, particularly in insulin users. Investigators are studying whether acarbose may be used one day as a substitute for that "morning insulin." The usual rules apply here: Acarbose should complement your meal plan and exercise routine; it is not a substitute or a way out, and does not, by itself, cause hypoglycemia.

Who Should Take Acarbose?

Acarbose is recommended for the following patients:

- Anyone who cannot control his or her blood sugar through diet and lifestyle modification alone.
- Anyone who is on OHAs but is still experiencing high blood sugar levels after meals.
- Anyone who cannot take OHAs and in whom diet/lifestyle modification has failed.
- Anyone not doing well on an OHA, who wants to prevent the advent of starting insulin treatment.

Who Should Not Take Acarbose?

Anyone with the following conditions should not be taking this drug:

- Inflammation or ulceration of the bowel (inflammatory bowel disease, ulcerative colitis, or Crohn's disease).
- Any kind of bowel obstruction.
- Any gastrointestinal disease.
- Kidney or liver disorders.
- Hernias.
- Pregnancy or lactation.
- Type 1 diabetes.

Dosage

The usual starting dosage for acarbose is 25 mg (half of a 50-mg tablet), with the first bite of each main meal. After four to eight weeks, your dosage may be increased to 50 mg, three times a day. Or you may start by taking one 50-mg tablet once daily with supper. If that's not working, you'll move up to two 50-mg tablets twice daily with your main meals or three 50-mg tablets three times daily with main meals. The maximum dosage of acarbose shouldn't go beyond 100 mg three times a day.

For best results, it's crucial that you take acarbose with the first bite of each main meal. In fact, if you swallow your pill even five to ten minutes before a meal, acarbose will pass through your digestive system and have no effect. It's also important that you take acarbose with a carbohydrate; the medication doesn't work if there are no carbohydrates in your meal. You shouldn't take acarbose between meals, either; it won't work. Nor should acarbose be used as a weight loss drug.

Side Effects

The good news is that acarbose doesn't cause hypoglycemia. Since you may be taking this drug along with an OHA, however, you may still experience hypoglycemia, as acarbose doesn't prevent it, either. The only side effects acarbose, by itself, causes are gastrointestinal: gas, abdominal cramps, soft stools, or diarrhea. Acarbose combined with Metformin, though, can produce unacceptable gastrointestinal symptoms. You'll notice these side effects after you've consumed foods that contain lots of sugar. Avoid taking antacids; they won't be effective in this case. Adjusting the dosage and making sure you're taking acarbose correctly will usually take care of side effects.

34. Ask About Thiazoladinediones

Thiazoladinediones are pills that make your cells more sensitive to insulin, thereby improving insulin resistance. When this happens, more glucose gets into your tissues and less glucose hangs around in your blood. The result is that you'll have lower fasting blood glucose levels, without the need to increase insulin levels. Both Avandia (rosiglitazone) and Actos (pioglitazone) work by stimulating muscle tissue to "drink in" glucose. They also decrease glucose production from the liver and make fat tissue more receptive to glucose. These drugs are reserved for people with Type 2 diabetes who must take insulin to reduce their blood sugar levels.

The first thiazoladinedione drug, Rezulin (troglitazone), was taken off the market in March 2000 because of the high risk of severe liver damage or liver failure associated with it. In early studies done with Rezulin, only 1.9 percent of people in the trial developed mild liver problems. But as soon as the drug was more widely prescribed, the U.S. Food and Drug Administration received reports of several cases of severe liver disease that led to death or the need for a liver transplant. For example, in one case, a fifty-five-year-old woman using insulin who took a daily dose of 400 mg of troglitazone for about three months developed liver failure. Avandia and Actos, both released in 1999, are very similar in chemical structure to Rezulin, but seem to have a much lower risk of liver damage than Rezulin. Nevertheless, it's very important to ask your doctor about the risks of either drug if they are prescribed. If you've ever had hepatitis (A, B, or C), you should not take this drug. There are a number of other factors in your history that may prevent you from being on the drug, which you must discuss with your doctor.

The average starting dose for Avandia is 4 mg per day, but doses range from 2 to 8 mg. The starting dose for Actos is either 15 mg or 30 mg per day, with a maximum dosage of 45 mg per day.

Other Side Effects

Trials with Rezulin showed that anyone with cardiovascular problems, or who was immune suppressed for any reason, should not be on it. Therefore, it's important to discuss the risks of Avandia or Actos with your doctor if you have cardiovascular problems or are immune suppressed, since the chemical structure of these drugs is similar to Rezulin.

35. Know the Natural Alternatives

If you don't like the idea of taking pills to control your diabetes, you can try to incorporate more natural methods to see if you can prevent taking medication. You'll have to discuss this approach with your doctor, of course, but here are some options:

- Guar gum. This is a great source of fiber, made from the seeds of the Indian cluster bean. When you mix guar with water, it turns into a gummy gel, which slows down your digestive system, similar in effect to acarbose (see page 70). Guar is often used as a natural treatment for high blood sugar as well as high cholesterol. Guar can cause gas, stomachaches, nausea, and diarrhea. (These are also side effects of acarbose.) The problem with guar is that there are no scientific studies to date concluding that it improves blood sugar control. Nevertheless, most experts agree that it can certainly provide some marginal benefits.

- Delay glucose absorption by eating more fiber, avoiding table sugar (sucrose), and eating small meals more often to space out your calories.

36. Know the Questions to Ask About Diabetes Drugs

Before you fill your prescription, it's important to ask your doctor or pharmacist the following:

1. What does this drug contain? If you are allergic to particular ingredients, such as dyes, it's important to find out the drug's ingredients before you take it.

2. Are there any medications I shouldn't combine with this drug? Be sure to ask about interactions with cholesterol or hypertension medications, as well as with any antidepressants or antipsychotics.

3. If this drug doesn't work well, am I a candidate for combination therapy? This means that your drug could be combined with another drug. Common "combo platters" are a sulphonylurea and biguanide, or acarbose and an OHA. Either the first drug you started is raised to its maximum dosage, before the second drug is started at its lowest dosage, or both drugs are started at their lowest dosages and then raised gradually.

4. If this drug doesn't work well, would insulin ever be prescribed along with this pill? It remains controversial whether combining insulin with a pill does any good. Nevertheless, some studies have shown that there is some benefit.

5. How will you measure the effectiveness of my drug? You should be testing your blood sugar with a glucose monitor, particularly two hours after eating, to make sure that the lowest effective dose can be prescribed. Your doctor should also be doing a glycosylated hemoglobin (HbA1c) test two to three times per year (as discussed earlier).

6. How should I store my drugs? All pills should be kept in a dry place at a temperature between 15°C and 25°C. Keep these drugs away from children, don't give them out as "samples" to your sister-in-law, and don't use tablets beyond their expiration date.

7. What symptoms should I watch out for while on these drugs? You'll definitely want to watch for signs of high or low blood sugar.

37. Know When You Need to Take Insulin

Right now, 40 to 50 percent of all people with Type 2 diabetes require insulin injections to manage their condition. Let me dispel a common fear about insulin: Since insulin is not a blood product, you don't have to worry about being infected with a blood-borne virus such as HIV or hepatitis. Many doctors often delay insulin therapy for as long as possible by giving you maximum doses of the pills discussed earlier. This is not good diabetes management; if you need insulin, you should take insulin. The goal is to get your disease under control. Therefore, anyone with the following conditions is a candidate for insulin:

- High blood sugar levels, despite maximum doses of oral hypoglycemic agents.

- Fasting glucose levels consistently over 162 mg/dl (9 mmol/L).

- Illness or stress (insulin may be needed until you recover).

- Major surgery.

- Complications of diabetes. (See Part Five.)

- Pregnancy (insulin may be temporary).

If going on insulin will affect your job security, you should discuss this with your doctor so that appropriate notes or letters can be drafted to those concerned. You should also keep in mind that if insulin therapy does not bring your diabetes under control within six months of treatment, it may be necessary to return to your drug therapy, after all.

The Right Insulin

The goal of a good insulin program is to try to mimic what your pancreas would do if it were working properly. Blood sugar rises in a sort of wave pattern. The big waves come in after a big meal; the small waves come in after a small meal or snack. The insulin program needs to be matched to your own particular wave pattern. So what you eat—and when—has a lot to do with the correct insulin program. Therefore, the right insulin for someone who eats three square meals a day may not be appropriate for someone who tends to graze all day. And the right insulin for an active forty-seven-year-old man in a stressful job may not be the right insulin for a sixty-seven-year-old woman who does not work and whose heart condition prevents her from exercising regularly.

You and your health care team also must decide how much control you need over your blood sugar. Insulin "recipes" depend on whether you need tight control (3 to 6 mmol), medium control (4 to 10 mmol/L), or even loose control (11 to 13 mmol/L). Loose control is certainly not encouraged, but in rare circumstances, when a person is quite elderly and suffering from a number of other health problems, for example, it is still practiced. To determine the appropriate insulin recipe for you, your health care team should look at who you are as a person—what you eat, where you work (do you work shifts?), your willingness to change your eating habits, and other lifestyle factors.

There are many kinds of insulin available. Every manufacturer has a different brand name of insulin and a separate letter code for the insulin action. See Item 39 for more details.

38. Get to Know Your Insulin

Use the guidelines that follow to identify and learn about what kind of insulin you've been prescribed. For information about brand names, premixed insulins, and specific products, consult your doctor, pharmacist, diabetes educator, or insulin manufacturer.

Short-Acting Insulin

(This is the "hare." It gets there fast but tires easily.)

- Starts working: in thirty minutes (Insulin Lispro: less than fifteen to thirty minutes).
- Peak effect: two to four hours (Insulin Lispro: thirty minutes to two-and-a-half hours).

- Duration of action: six to eight hours (Insulin Lispro: three to four hours).
- When to eat: within thirty minutes of injecting.
- Exits body: in eight hours.
- Appearance: clear. Don't use if cloudy, or slightly colored or if solid chunks are visible.

Intermediate-Acting Insulin

(This is the "tortoise." It gets there at a slower pace, but it lasts longer.)

- Starts working: one to two hours.
- Peak effect: four to twelve hours (usually around eight or less).
- Duration of action: twenty-four hours (or less).
- When to eat: within two hours.
- Exits body: in twenty-four hours.
- Appearance: cloudy. Do not use if the white material remains at the bottom of the bottle after mixing, leaving a clear liquid above; or if clumps are floating in the insulin after mixing; or if it has a frosted appearance.

Long-Acting Insulin

(This is the "two-legged turtle." It's really slow, and it hangs around for a long time.)

- Starts working: in eight hours.
- Peak effect: in eighteen hours.
- Duration of action: thirty-six hours.

- When to eat: within eight hours.
- Exits body: in thirty-six hours or more.
- Appearance: cloudy. Do not use if the white material remains at the bottom of the bottle after mixing, leaving a clear liquid above; or if clumps are floating in the insulin after mixing; or if it has a frosted appearance.

39. Know Your Insulin Codes

This list is a code breaker that will help you identify exactly what kind of insulin you're taking.

R: This stands for regular biosynthetic human insulin. Regular means that it is short-acting insulin.

"ge" Toronto: "ge" is the name Connaught-Novo gives to all its biosynthetic insulin. It stands for genetically engineered. Toronto is the brand name of this company's short-acting insulin, like Kraft or President's Choice.

Insulin Lispro: This is a very new and super-short acting insulin sold under the brand name Humalog. It starts to work in fifteen to thirty minutes. It is a biosynthetic insulin made from two amino acids, LYS and PRO. It's ideal for people with Type 1 diabetes.

N or NPH: NPH are the initials of the man who invented this type of insulin, which is an intermediate-acting insulin that is said to have an abrupt peak. ("ge"-NPH stands for genetically engineered NPH.)

L or Lente: This is also an intermediate-acting insulin that is very similar to NPH except it has a more gradual peak. ("ge"-Lente stands for genetically engineered Lente.)

Beef/Pork: This is animal insulin made from cows or pigs. It's still available from Eli Lilly but isn't readily available at most pharmacies unless it's special ordered.

Humulin 10/90: This is a premixed insulin, meaning that it is 10 percent regular and 90 percent NPH. Also available in 20/80, 30/70, 40/60, and 50/50. (Note: Many people with Type 2 diabetes do well on 30/70.)

Novolin 10/90 "ge": Exactly the same as above, except "ge," which stands for genetically engineered, the label Connaught-Novo gives to its biosynthetic insulin.

Novolin ultra "ge": Connaught-Novo's long-acting insulin, which starts acting in four hours, peaks within eight to twenty-four hours, and exits within twenty-eight hours. Again, "ge" stands for genetically engineered.

Ultra Lente "ge": The same as above except it peaks in ten to thirty hours and exits in thirty-six hours.

Semi Lente-NPH: This is a very long-acting insulin that is rarely used. Most diabetes educators haven't seen someone on this stuff for years!

40. Learn How to Use Insulin Properly

Once you and your diabetes health care team choose the right insulin for you, you will need to have a minicourse on how to use and inject insulin. This is usually done by a certified diabetes educator (CDE).

Your Insulin Gear

If you've graduated to insulin therapy, here's what you'll need to buy:

- A really good glucose monitor that is made for people who test frequently.
- Lancets and a lancing device for testing your blood sugar.
- Insulin pens and cartridges (this is far easier) or traditional needles and syringes (a diabetes educator needs to walk you through the types of products available).
- The right insulin brand for you.

Insulin must be injected. It cannot be taken orally because your own stomach acids digest the insulin before it has a chance to work. Your doctor, pharmacist, CDE, or someone at a diabetes care center will teach you how to inject yourself painlessly. Don't inject insulin by yourself without a training session. The most convenient way to use insulin is with an insulin pen. In this case, your insulin (if human or biosynthetic) will come in a cartridge. If you decide against a pen, your insulin will come in a bottle, and you will need a needle and syringe. Always know the answers to these questions before you inject your insulin:

- How long does it take before it starts to work? (Known as the onset of action.)
- When is this insulin working the hardest? (Known as the peak.)
- How long will my insulin continue to work? (Known as the duration of action.)

How Many Injections Will I Need?

This really depends on what kind of insulin you're taking and why you're taking it. A sample routine may be to take an injection in the morning, a second injection before supper, and a third before bed. What you want to prevent is low blood sugar while you're sleeping. You may need to adjust your insulin if there is a change in your food or exercise routine (which could happen if you're sick). Your insulin schedule is usually carefully matched to your meal times and exercise periods.

Where to Inject Insulin

The good news is that you do not have to inject insulin into a vein. As long as it makes it under your skin or in a muscle, you're fine. Thighs and tummies are popular injection sites. These are also large enough areas that you can vary your injection site. (You should space your injections about 2 to 3 cm apart.) Usually you establish a little rotating pattern. Other injection sites are the upper outer area of the arms, the upper outer surfaces of the buttocks, and the lower back area.

Insulin injected in the abdomen is absorbed more quickly than insulin injected in the thigh. In addition, strenuous exercise will speed up the rate of its absorption if the insulin is injected into the limb you've just exercised. Other factors that can affect insulin's action are the depth of injection, your dose, the temperature (it should be room temperature or body temperature), and what animal your insulin came from (human, cow, or pig).

Experts also suggest you massage the injection site to increase the rate of insulin absorption. If your skin hardens due to overuse, this will affect the rate of absorption. Your doctor or CDE will show you how to actually inject your insulin (angles, pinching folds of skin, and so on). There are lots of tricks of the trade to optimize comfort. With the fine needle points available today, insulin use doesn't have to be an uncomfortable ordeal.

Side Effects

The main side effect of insulin therapy is low blood sugar, which means that you must eat or drink glucose to combat symptoms. This side effect is also known as insulin shock. You may also notice something called lipodystrophy (a change in the fatty tissue under the skin) or hypertrophy (an enlarged area on your skin). Rotating your injection sites will prevent these problems. A sunken area on the skin surface may also appear, but is usually only present with animal insulin. Rashes can sometimes occur at injection sites, too. Less than 5 percent of all insulin users notice these problems, however.

Questions to Ask About Insulin

The answers to these questions depend on your insulin brand. Pharmacists and doctors should know the answers to all these questions, but if they don't, I recommend calling the customer care toll-free number provided by your insulin manufacturer.

- How do I store this insulin?
- What are the characteristics of this insulin (that is, onset of action, peak, and duration of action)?

- When should I eat after injecting this insulin?
- When should I exercise after injecting this insulin?
- How long are opened insulin bottles/cartridges safe at room temperature?
- What about the effect of sunlight or extreme temperatures on this insulin?
- Should this insulin be shaken or rolled?
- What should I do if the insulin sticks to the inside of the vial/cartridge?
- Should this insulin be clear or cloudy? What should I do if the appearance looks "off" or has changed?
- What happens if I accidentally inject out-of-date insulin?
- What other medications can interfere with this particular brand?
- Who should I see about switching insulin brands?
- If I've switched from animal to human insulin, what dose should I be on?

Traveling with Insulin

When traveling, you'll need to make sure you pack enough insulin for your trip, as well as identification (such as a doctor's note) that clearly states you have diabetes, so you don't get harassed over carrying needles, syringes, and vials. In fact, many experts suggest that for a trip, you switch to an insulin pen, which is far easier to carry and less obvious. In some cases, even lancets and a glucose meter may be suspect without identification. Experts recommend the following supplies for travel:

- A backup supply of insulin you keep with you, as well as extra cartridges, needles, syringes, and testing supplies; vials break, baggage gets lost, and planes, trains, and buses get delayed.

- A doctor's written prescription for your insulin and a doctor's note explaining why you're carrying your equipment.

- A MedicAlert tag or card stating that you have diabetes.

- A day's supply of food (especially if you're flying).

- An extra sugar source, such as dextrose tablets.

- A list of hospitals in your travel destination areas.

It's important never to part with your insulin; always carry it with you in carry-on baggage. Dividing your supplies between two bags is best in case vials break. If you're flying, drink lots of liquids prior to boarding, as well as one glass of nonalcoholic liquid for every hour of flight. And don't order a special meal; these have a nasty habit of never making it to your plane. Bring food with you and pick at the plane food you're served. You should also stroll up and down the cabin as much as possible to avoid high blood sugar. (This bit of exercise will use up some sugar.) If you're traveling to a different time zone, consult your doctor or diabetes educator about adjusting insulin injections to the new time zone.

PART FIVE

Preventing Complications

41. Remember the Ultimate Goal of Managing Type 2 Diabetes

Why is it so important to manage your diabetes? Because many of the preexisting conditions that led to your diabetes can cause other complications down the road. On top of that, walking around with higher-than-normal blood sugar levels can lead to even more complications.

At least 40 percent of all people with Type 2 will develop another disease as a result of their diabetes. Many of you reading this may already be affected by some of the conditions discussed in the upcoming pages. But if you've been newly diagnosed with Type 2 diabetes, you may not realize exactly how many other diseases can be triggered by it; after all, you may feel fine now. The purpose of the information that follows is to simplify the complicated language of "complications," so you can see what's possible down the road, clearly read the road signs, and perhaps takes a different route. You'll find out why diabetes leads to other diseases, the diagnosis and treatment of each of those diseases, and what can be done to prevent complications.

42. Understand Macrovascular Versus Microvascular Complications

The most important thing to grasp about diabetes complications is that there are two kinds of problems that can lead to similar diseases. The first kind of problem is known as a macrovascular complication. The prefix *macro* means large, as in macroeconomics (studying an entire economic system as opposed to one company's economic structure). The word *vascular* means blood vessels—your veins and arteries, which carry the blood back and forth throughout your body. Put these together and you have "large blood vessel complications." But a plain-language interpretation of macrovascular complications would be, "big problems with your blood vessels."

If you think of your body as a planet, a macrovascular disease would be a disease that affects the whole planet; it is bodywide, or systemic. Cardiovascular disease is a macrovascular complication that can cause heart attack, stroke, high blood pressure, and bodywide circulation problems, clinically known as peripheral vascular disease (PVD). So your body—head to toe—is affected.

A second type of problem is known as a microvascular complication. *Micro* means tiny, as in microscopic. Microvascular complications refer to problems with the small blood vessels (capillaries) that connect to various body parts. A plain-language interpretation of microvascular complications would be, "Houston, we've got a problem." In other words, the problem is serious, but it's not going to affect the whole planet, just the spacecraft in orbit. Eye disease (clinically known as retinopathy) is a microvascular complication. Blindness is a serious problem, but you won't die from it. Nerve damage (neuropathy) is a microvascular complication that can affect your whole body—feet, eyes, sexual functioning, skin—but, again, you won't die from it.

Here's where complications get really complicated to understand: when macro and micro converge. This is what happens with kidney disease (clinically known as renal disease nephropathy). The high blood pressure that is caused by macrovascular complications, combined with the small blood vessel damage caused by microvascular complications, together can cause kidney failure—something you can die from unless you have dialysis (filtering out the body's waste products through a machine) or a kidney transplant.

43. Know Who Gets Macrovascular Complications

Macrovascular complications are caused not only by too much blood sugar but also by preexisting health problems. People with Type 2 diabetes are far more vulnerable to macrovascular complications because they usually have contributing risk factors from way back, such as high cholesterol and high blood pressure. Obesity, smoking, and inactivity can then aggravate those problems, resulting in major cardiovascular disease.

Warning Signs of Macrovascular Complications

If you are obese, inactive, and have Type 2 diabetes as well as high blood pressure and/or high cholesterol—these are the warning signs of macrovascular problems. The bomb is ticking. In this case, you should work right now on making changes in your diet and lifestyle and discuss with your doctor whether you're a candidate for blood pressure–lowering or cholesterol-lowering medication. If you're a woman entering menopause, you should definitely consider hormone replacement therapy, which offers protection from heart disease, balancing the benefits of that against other risks. You may also want to look into more effective strategies to manage your obesity.

You also need to stay alert to signs of circulation problems, heart attack, and stroke, which are discussed in detail further on.

44. Know Who Gets Microvascular Complications

People with Type 1 diabetes are very vulnerable to microvascular complications, but a good portion of people with Type 2 diabetes suffer from them, too. Microvascular complications are known as sugar-related complications. Small blood vessel damage is caused by high blood sugar levels over long periods of time. The Diabetes Control and Complications Trial, discussed in detail in Item 50, showed that by keeping blood sugar levels as normal as possible, as often as possible, through frequent self-testing, microvascular complications can be prevented.

Warning Signs of Microvascular Problems

Numbness in arms, face, or legs, vision problems, bladder infections, and other bladder difficulties are warning signs of microvascular problems. Specific alarm signals for each microvascular problem are discussed separately further on.

45. Know Your Risk of Heart Attack or Stroke

Type 2 diabetes is often called "a heart attack about to happen." When large blood vessels are damaged, it means cardiovascular disease (heart disease). The first sign of heart disease is angina, or chest pains. When blood vessels get blocked due to hardening of the arteries (clinically known as arteriosclerosis), not enough blood gets to the heart muscle, causing it to die. That's what a heart attack is.

Peripheral vascular disease (meaning "fringe" blood-flow problems) is part of the heart disease story. PVD occurs when blood flow to the limbs (arms, legs, and feet) is blocked, which creates cramping, pains, or numbness. In fact, pain and numbness in your arms or legs may be signs of heart disease or even an imminent heart attack.

The way to prevent heart disease and peripheral vascular disease is by modifying your lifestyle (stop smoking, eat less fat, get more exercise). Blood pressure–lowering medication and cholesterol-lowering drugs are also an option if you have high blood pressure and/or high cholesterol. And, finally, heart surgery, which includes angioplasty, laser treatment, and bypass surgery is an option. Smoking, high blood pressure, high blood sugar, and high cholesterol (called the catastrophic quartet by one diabetes specialist) will greatly increase your risk of heart disease.

Cardiovascular disease puts you at risk for a stroke, which occurs when a blood clot (a clog in your blood vessels) travels to your brain and stops the flow of blood and oxygen carried to the nerve cells in that area. When that happens, cells may die or vital functions controlled by the brain can be temporarily or permanently damaged.

Bleeding or a rupture from the affected blood vessel can lead to very serious complications, including death. People with Type 2 diabetes are two to three times more likely to suffer from a stroke than people without diabetes.

Since the 1960s, the death rate from strokes has dropped by 50 percent. This drop is largely due to public awareness campaigns regarding diet and lifestyle modification (quitting smoking, eating low-fat foods, and exercising), as well as the introduction of blood pressure–lowering drugs and cholesterol-lowering medications that have helped people maintain normal blood pressure and cholesterol levels.

Strokes can be mild, moderate, severe, or fatal. Mild strokes may affect speech or movement for a short period of time only; many people recover from mild strokes without any permanent damage. Moderate or severe strokes may result in loss of speech and memory, and paralysis; many people learn to speak again and learn to function with partial paralysis. How well you recover depends on how much damage is done. It's never too late to reduce the risk of stroke by quitting smoking and making even small changes in diet and lifestyle. Discuss with your doctor whether you're a candidate for medications that can control your blood pressure and cholesterol levels. Aiming for normal blood sugar levels as often as possible is also important. A considerable amount of research points to stress as a risk factor for stroke.

Signs of a Stroke

If you can recognize the key warning signs of a stroke, it can make a difference in preventing a major stroke or in the severity of a stroke.

Call 911 or get to an emergency room if you suddenly notice one or more of the following symptoms:

- Weakness, numbness, and/or tingling in your face, arms, or legs. (This may last only a few moments.)
- Loss of speech or difficulty understanding somebody else's speech. (This may last only a short time.)
- Severe headaches that feel different than any headache you've had before.
- Feeling unsteady or falling a lot.

46. Know Your Risk of Nerve Disease

When your blood sugar levels are too high for too long, you can develop a condition known as diabetic neuropathy, or nerve disease. Somehow, the cells that make up your nerves are altered in response to high blood sugar. This condition can lead to foot amputation in people with diabetes.

There are different groups of nerves that are affected by high blood sugar; keeping your blood sugar levels as normal as possible is the best way to prevent many of the following problems. Drugs that help to prevent chemical changes in your nerve cells can also be used to treat nerve damage. The following nerve diseases can develop:

Polyneuropathy is a disease that affects the nerves in your feet and legs. The symptoms are burning, tingling, and numbness in the legs and feet.

Autonomic neuropathy is a disease that affects the nerves you don't notice; the nerves that control your digestive tract, blood pressure, sweat glands, overall balance, and sexual functioning. Treatment varies depending on what's affected, but there are drugs that can control individual parts of the body, such as the digestive tract.

Proximal motor neuropathy is a disease that affects the nerves that control your muscles. This can lead to weakness and burning sensations in the joints (hands, thighs, and ankles are the most common). These problems can be individually treated with physiotherapy and/or specific medication. When the nerves that control the muscles in the eyes are affected, you may experience problems with your eyesight, such as double vision. Finally, nerve damage can affect the spine, causing pain and loss of sensation in the back, buttocks, and legs.

47. Know How to Protect Your Eyes

Diabetes is the leading cause of new blindness in adults. Seventy-eight percent of people with Type 2 diabetes experience diabetes eye disease, clinically known as diabetic retinopathy. Microvascular complications damage the small blood vessels in the eyes. High blood pressure, associated with macrovascular complications, also damages the blood vessels in the eyes.

While 98 percent of people with Type 1 diabetes will experience eye disease within fifteen years of being diagnosed, in Type 2 diabetes, eye disease is often diagnosed before the diabetes; in other words, many people don't realize they have diabetes until their eye doctors ask them, "Have you been screened for diabetes?" In fact, 20 percent of people with Type 2 diabetes already have diabetes eye disease before their diabetes is diagnosed.

What Happens to the Eyes?

Eighty percent of all eye disease is known as nonproliferative eye disease, meaning "no new blood vessel growth" eye disease. This is also called background diabetic eye disease. In this case, the blood vessels in the retina (the part of your eyeball that faces your brain, as opposed to your face) start to deteriorate, bleed, or hemorrhage (known as microaneurysms) and leak water and protein into the center of the retina, called the macula; this condition is known as macular edema, and causes vision loss, which sometimes is only temporary. Without treatment, however, more permanent vision loss will occur.

Proliferative eye disease means "new blood vessel growth" eye disease. In this case, your retina says, "Since all my blood vessels are being damaged, I'm just going to grow new blood vessels!" This process is known as neovascularization. The problem is that these new blood vessels are deformed, or abnormal, which makes the situation worse, not better. These deformed blood vessels look a bit like Swiss cheese; they're full of holes and have a bad habit of suddenly bleeding out, causing severe damage without warning. They can also lead to scar tissue in the retina, retinal detachments, and glaucoma, greatly increasing the risk of legal blindness.

Symptoms

In the early stages of diabetes eye disease, there are no symptoms. That's why you need to have a thorough eye exam every six months. As eye damage progresses, you may notice blurred vision. The blurred vision is due to changes in the shape of the lens of the eye. During an eye exam, your ophthalmologist may notice yellow spots on your retina, signs that scar tissue has formed on the retina from bleeding. If the disease progresses to the point where new blood vessels have formed, vision problems may be quite severe, as a result of spontaneous bleeding or detachment of the retina. Other diabetes-related eye problems that may affect vision include cataracts and glaucoma, as previously mentioned.

How to Protect Yourself from Diabetes Eye Disease

Early detection is your best protection! Using Type 1 rules is the best way to detect diabetes eye disease early and prevent vision loss. In other words, it's crucial to have frequent eye exams. Teens or young adults diagnosed with Type 1 diabetes should have semiannual or annual eye exams. This way, eye disease can be detected before it affects vision permanently. The average person has an eye exam every five years. And if you're walking around with undiagnosed Type 2 diabetes, you can also be walking around with early signs of diabetes eye disease. So as soon as you're diagnosed with Type 2 diabetes, get to an eye specialist for a complete exam and make it a yearly "gig" from now on.

During an eye exam, an ophthalmologist will dilate your pupil with eyedrops, and then use a special instrument to check for:

- Tiny red dots (signs of bleeding).
- A thick or milky retina, with or without yellow clumps or spots (signs of macular edema).

- A "bathtub ring" on the retina—a ring shape that surrounds a leakage site on the retina (also a sign of macular edema).

- "Cottonwool spots" on the retina—small, fluffy white patches on the retina (signs of new blood vessel growth, or more advanced eye disease).

Today, it's estimated that if everyone with impaired glucose tolerance went for an eye exam once a year, blindness from diabetes eye disease would drop from 8 percent in this group to 1 percent.

Can Diabetes Eye Disease Be Treated?

Diabetes eye disease is not completely treatable. A procedure known as laser photocoagulation can burn and seal off the damaged blood vessels, which stops them from bleeding or leaking. In the earlier stages of eye disease, this procedure can restore your vision within about six months. In most cases, however, laser surgery only slows down vision loss, rather than restoring vision. In other words, without the treatment, your vision will get worse; with the treatment, it will stay the same.

If new blood vessels have already formed, a series of laser treatments are used to purposely scar the retina. Since a scarred retina needs less oxygen, blood vessels stop re-forming, reducing the risk of further damage. In more serious cases, surgery known as a *vitrectomy* is performed. In this procedure, blood and scar tissue on the retina are surgically removed.

If you're suffering from vision loss, a number of visual aids can help you perform daily tasks more easily. Your doctor or diabetes educator can refer you to sources of these aids.

A Word About Smoking

Since smoking also damages blood vessels, and diabetes eye disease is a blood vessel disease, smoking will certainly aggravate the problem. Quitting smoking may help to reduce eye complications. Not everyone can quit smoking cold turkey, although it's a strategy that many have used successfully. (Some cold turkey quitters report that keeping one package of cigarettes within reach lessens anxiety.) The symptoms of nicotine withdrawal begin within a few hours and peak at twenty-four to forty-eight hours after quitting. You may experience anxiety, irritability, hostility, restlessness, insomnia, and anger. For these reasons, many smokers turn to smoking cessation programs, which can include any of the following:

- Behavioral counseling: Behavioral counseling, either group or individual, can raise the rate of abstinence to 20 to 25 percent. This approach to smoking cessation aims to change the mental processes of smoking, reinforce the benefits of nonsmoking, and teach skills to help the smoker avoid the urge to smoke.

- Nicotine gum: Nicotine gum (Nicorette) is now available over the counter. It works as an aid to help you quit smoking by reducing nicotine cravings and withdrawal symptoms. Nicotine gum helps you wean yourself from nicotine by allowing you to gradually decrease the dosage until you stop using it altogether, a process which usually takes about twelve weeks. The only disadvantage with this method is that it caters to the oral and addictive aspects of smoking (rewarding the urge to smoke with a dose of nicotine).

- Nicotine patch: Transdermal nicotine, or the "patch" (Habitrol, Nicoderm, Nicotrol), doubles abstinence rates in former smokers. Most brands are now available over the counter. Each morning, a new patch is applied to a different area of dry, clean, hairless skin and left on for the day. Some patches are designed to be worn a full twenty-four hours. The constant supply of nicotine to the bloodstream sometimes causes very vivid or disturbing dreams, however. You can also expect to feel a mild itching, burning, or tingling at the site of the patch when it is first applied. The nicotine patch works best when it is worn for at least seven to twelve weeks, with a gradual decrease in strength (nicotine). Many smokers find it effective because it allows them to tackle the psychological addiction to smoking before they are forced to deal with physical symptoms of withdrawal.

- Nicotine inhaler: The nicotine inhaler (Nicotrol Inhaler) delivers nicotine orally via inhalation from a plastic tube. Its success rate is about 28 percent, similar to that of nicotine gum. It's available by prescription only in the United States. Like nicotine gum, the inhaler mimics smoking behavior by responding to each craving or urge to smoke, a feature that has both advantages and disadvantages to the smoker who wants to get over the physical symptoms of withdrawal. The nicotine inhaler should be used for a period of twelve weeks.

- Nicotine nasal spray: Like nicotine gum and the nicotine patch, the nasal spray reduces craving and withdrawal symptoms, allowing smokers to cut back gradually. One squirt delivers about 1 mg nicotine. In three clinical trials involving 730 patients, 31 to 35 percent were not smoking at six months. This compares to an average of 12 to 15 percent of smokers who were able to quit unaided. The nasal spray has a couple of advantages over the gum and the patch: Nicotine is rapidly absorbed across the nasal membranes, providing a kick that is more like the real thing; and the prompt onset of action plus a flexible dosing schedule benefits heavier smokers. Because the nicotine reaches your bloodstream so quickly, nasal sprays do have a greater potential for addiction than the slower acting gum and patch.

- Alternative therapies: Hypnosis, meditation, and acupuncture have helped some smokers quit. In the case of hypnosis and meditation, sessions may be private or part of a group smoking cessation program.

The drug bupropion (Zyban) is now available and is an option for people who have been unsuccessful using nicotine replacement. Formerly prescribed as an antidepressant, its other use was discovered by accident: Researchers knew that quitting smokers were often depressed, and so they began experimenting with the drug as a means to fight depression, not addiction. Bupropion reduces the withdrawal symptoms associated with smoking cessation and can be used in conjunction with nicotine replacement therapy. Researchers suspect that bupropion works directly in the brain to disrupt the addictive power of nicotine by affecting the same chemical neurotransmitters ("messengers") in the brain, such as dopamine, that nicotine does.

The pleasurable aspect of addictive drugs such as nicotine and cocaine is triggered by the release of dopamine. Smoking floods the brain with dopamine. *The New England Journal of Medicine* published the results of a study of more than six hundred smokers taking bupropion. At the end of treatment, 44 percent of those who took the highest dose of the drug (300 mg) were not smoking, compared to 19 percent of the group who took a placebo. By the end of one year, 23 percent of the 300-mg group and 12 percent of the placebo group were still smoke free. Using Zyban with nicotine replacement therapy seems to improve the quit rate a bit further. Four-week quit rates from the study were 23 percent for placebo, 36 percent for the patch, 49 percent for Zyban, and 58 percent for a combination of Zyban and the patch.

Eye Infections

High blood sugar can predispose you to frequent bacterial infections, including conjunctivitis (pinkeye). Eye infections can also affect your vision. To prevent eye infections, make sure you wash your hands before you touch your eyes, especially before you handle contact lenses.

48. Know How to Protect Your Feet

Foot complications related to diabetes were dramatized in the mid-1980s film *Nothing in Common*, in which Jackie Gleason plays the ne'er-do-well diabetic father, and Tom Hanks plays the son who cannot accept him. In a heartbreaking scene, Tom Hanks is shocked to discover how ill his father really is when he finally sees his feet. They are swollen, purple, and badly infected. Ultimately, the story ends with the father and son coming to terms as Gleason must undergo surgical amputation.

I share this example with you because many of us are used to ignoring and abusing our feet. We wear uncomfortable shoes, we pick at our calluses and blisters, we don't wear socks with our shoes, and so on. You can't do this anymore. Your feet are the targets of both macrovascular (large blood vessel) complications and microvascular (small blood vessel) complications. In the first case, peripheral vascular disease affects blood circulation to your feet. In the second place, the nerve cells to your feet, which control sensation, can be altered through microvascular complications. Nerve damage can also affect the foot's muscles and tendons, causing weakness and changes to the foot's shape.

The combination of poor circulation and no feeling in your feet means that you can sustain an injury to your feet and not know about it. For example, you might step on a piece of glass or badly stub your toe and not realize it. If an open wound becomes infected and you have poor circulation, the wound may not heal properly, infection could spread to the bone, or gangrene could develop. In this situation, amputation may be the only treatment. Or, without sensation or proper circulation in them, your feet could be far more vulnerable to frostbite or exposure than they would be otherwise.

Diabetes accounts for approximately half of all nonemergency amputations, but all experts agree that doing a foot self-exam every day (see below) can prevent most foot complications from becoming severe. Those at highest risk for foot problems are people who still smoke (smoking aggravates all diabetic complications), are overweight (more weight on the feet), are over age forty, or have had diabetes for more than ten years.

Signs of Foot Problems

The most common symptoms of foot complications are burning, tingling, or pain in your feet or legs. These are all signs of nerve damage. Numbness is another symptom, which could mean nerve damage or circulation problems. If you do experience pain from nerve damage, it usually gets worse with time (as new nerves and blood vessels grow), and many people find that it's worse at night. Bed linens can actually increase discomfort. Some people only notice foot symptoms after exercising or a short walk. But many people don't notice immediate symptoms until they've lost feeling in their feet.

Other symptoms people notice are frequent infections (caused by blood vessel damage), hair loss on the toes or lower legs, or shiny skin on the lower legs and feet.

When You Knock Your Socks Off

When you take off your socks at the end of the day, get in the habit of doing a foot self-exam. This is a good way to monitor your feet. You're looking for signs of infection or potential infection triggers. If you can avoid infection at all costs, you will be able to keep your feet. Look for the following signs:

- Reddened, discolored, or swollen areas (blue, bright red, or white areas mean that circulation is cut off).
- Pus.
- Temperature changes in the feet, or "hot spots."
- Corns, calluses, and warts. (Potential infections could be hiding under calluses; do not remove these yourself—see a podiatrist.)

- Toenails that are too long. (Your toenail could cut you if it's too long.)
- Redness where your shoes or socks are rubbing due to a poor fit. (When your sock is scrunched inside your shoe, the folds could actually rub against the skin and cause a blister.)
- Toenail fungus (under the nail).
- Fungus between the toes. (This is athlete's foot, common if you've been walking around barefoot in a public place.)
- Breaks in the skin (especially between your toes), or cracks, such as in calluses on the heels; this opens the door for bacteria.

If you find an infection, wash your feet carefully with soap and water; don't use alcohol. Then see your doctor or a podiatrist (a foot specialist) as soon as possible. If your foot is irritated but not yet infected (redness, for example, from poor-fitting shoes but no blister yet), simply avoid the irritant—the shoes—and it should clear up. If not, see your doctor. If you're overweight and have trouble inspecting your feet, get somebody else to check them for the signs listed above. In addition to doing a self-exam, see your doctor to have the circulation and reflexes in your feet checked four times a year.

Foot Rules to Live By

- Walk a little bit every day; this is a good way to improve blood flow and get a little exercise!
- Don't walk around barefoot; wear proper-fitting, clean cotton socks with your shoes daily, and get in the habit of wearing slippers around the house and shoes at the

beach. If you're swimming, wear some sort of shoe (plastic "jellies" or canvas running shoes). This doesn't mean you have to look like the geek who wears white sports socks with Greek sandals; there are lots of options. If it's cold out, wear woolen socks.

- Before you put on your shoes, shake them out in case your (grand)child's Lego piece, a piece of dry cat food, or a pebble is in there.

- Wash your feet and lower legs every day in lukewarm water with mild soap. Dry them really well, especially between the toes.

- Trim your toenails straight across to avoid ingrown nails. Don't pick off your nails.

- No more "bathroom surgery" on your feet, which may include puncturing blisters with needles or tweezers, shaving your calluses, and the hundreds of other crazy things people do with their feet (but never disclose to their spouses).

- Baby your feet. When the skin seems too moist, use baby powder or a foot powder your doctor or pharmacist recommends (especially between the toes). When your feet are too dry, moisturize them with a lotion recommended by your doctor or pharmacist. The reason is simple: Breaks in the skin happen if feet are too moist (such as between the toes) or too dry (such as cracking). Use a foot buffing pad on your calluses after bathing.

- When you're sitting down, feet should be flat on the floor. Sitting cross-legged or in crossed-legged variations can cut off your circulation—and frequently does in people without diabetes.

- Wear comfortable, proper-fitting footwear. See Exhibit 48.1 for tips about shoe shopping.

EXHIBIT 48.1 How to Shoe-Shop for Health

To save your feet, you may not be able to save on your next pair of shoes. These are your new shoe-shopping rules:

- Shoe-shop at the time of day when your feet are most swollen (such as in the afternoon). That way, you'll purchase a shoe that fits you under all conditions.

- Don't even think about high heels or any type of shoe that is not comfortable or that doesn't fit properly. Say goodbye to thongs. That strip between your toes can cause too much irritation.

- Buy leather; avoid shoes with the terms "man-made upper" or "man-made materials" on the label—this means the shoes are made of synthetic materials and your foot will not breathe. Cotton or canvas shoes are fine, as long as the insole is cotton, too. Man-made materials on the very bottom of the shoe are fine as long as the upper—the part of the shoe that touches your foot—is leather, cotton/canvas, or something breathable.

- Remember that leather does, indeed, stretch. When that happens, the shoe could become loose and cause blisters. On the other hand, if the shoe is too tight and the salesperson tells you the shoe will stretch, forget it. The shoe will destroy you in the first few hours of wear, which sort of "defeets" the purpose.

- If you lose all sensation and cannot feel whether the shoe is fitting, make sure you have a shoe salesperson fit you.

- Avoid shoes that have been on display. A variety of people try these shoes on; you never know what bacteria and fungi these previously tried on shoes harbor.

Treatment for Open Wounds on the Feet or Legs

To heal cuts, sores, or any open wound, your body normally manufactures macrophages, special white blood cells that fight infection, as well as special repair cells called fibroblasts. These "ambulance cells" need oxygen to live. If you have poor circulation, it's akin to an ambulance not making it to an accident scene in time because it gets caught in a long traffic jam.

When wounds don't heal, gangrene infections can set in. Until recently, amputating the infected limb was the only way to deal with gangrene. But there is a therapy available at several hospitals called hyperbaric oxygen therapy (HBO). The procedure involves placing you in an oxygen chamber or tank and feeding you triple the amount of oxygen you'd find in the normal atmosphere. To heal gangrene on the feet, you'd need about thirty treatments (several per day for a week or so). The result is that your tissues become saturated with oxygen, enabling the body to heal itself. In one research trial, 89 percent of diabetics with foot gangrene were healed, compared to 1 percent of the control group. This treatment sounds expensive, but it's much cheaper than surgery, which is why HBO is catching on.

Not everybody is an HBO candidate; and not everybody has access to this therapy. But if you're being considered for surgical amputation, you should definitely ask about HBO first.

49. Know Your Risk of Kidney Disease

Both micro- and macrovascular complications can lead to kidney problems. High blood pressure and high blood sugar can be a dangerous combination for your kidneys. About 15 percent of people with Type 2 diabetes will develop kidney disease, known as either renal disease or nephropathy. In fact, diabetes causes 40 percent of all end-stage renal disease (ESRD), or kidney failure. Roughly 40 percent of all dialysis patients have diabetes.

What Do Your Kidneys Do All Day?

Kidneys are the public servants of the body; they're busy little bees! If they go on strike, you lose your water service, garbage pickup, and a few other services you don't even appreciate.

Kidneys regulate your body's water levels; when you have too much water, your kidneys remove it by dumping it into a large storage tank—your bladder. The excess water stays there until you're ready to urinate. If you don't have enough water in your body (or if you're dehydrated), your kidneys will retain the water for you to keep you balanced.

Kidneys also act as your body's sewage filtration plant. They filter out all the garbage and waste that your body doesn't need and dump it into the bladder; this waste is then excreted into your urine. The two waste products your kidneys regularly dump are urea (the waste product of protein) and creatinine (waste products produced by the muscles). In people with high blood sugar levels, excess sugar is sent to the kidneys, and the kidneys will dump it into the bladder, too, causing sugar to appear in the urine.

Kidneys also balance calcium and phosphate in the body, needed to build bones. Kidneys operate two little side businesses on top of all of this: they make two hormones. One hormone, called renin, helps to regulate blood pressure. Another hormone, called erythropoetin, helps bone marrow make red blood cells.

The Macro Thing

When you suffer from cardiovascular disease, you probably have high blood pressure. High blood pressure damages blood vessels in the kidneys, which interferes with their job performance. As a result, they won't be as efficient at removing waste or excess water from your body. And if you are experiencing poor circulation, which can also cause water retention, the problem is further aggravated.

Poor circulation may cause your kidneys to secrete too much renin, which is normally designed to regulate blood pressure, but in this case, increases it. All the extra fluid and the high blood pressure places a heavy burden on your heart—and your kidneys. If this situation isn't brought under control, you'd likely suffer from a heart attack before kidney failure, but kidney failure is inevitable.

The Micro Thing

When high blood sugar levels affect the small blood vessels, this includes the small blood vessels in the kidney's filters (called the nephrons). This condition is known as diabetic nephropathy. In the early stages of nephropathy, good, usable protein is secreted in the urine. That's a sign that the kidneys are unable to distribute usable protein to the body's tissues. (Normally, they would excrete only the waste product of protein—urea—into the urine.)

Another microvascular problem affects the kidneys: nerve damage. The nerves you use to control your bladder can be affected, causing a sort of sewage backup in your body. The first place that sewage hits is your kidneys. Old urine floating around your kidneys isn't a healthy thing. The kidneys can become damaged as a result, aggravating all the conditions we have discussed so far.

The Infection Thing

There's a third problem at work here. If you recall, frequent urination is a sign of high blood sugar. That's because your kidneys help to rid the body of too much sugar by dumping it into the bladder. Well, guess what? You're not the only one who likes sugar; bacteria, such as *e. coli* (the "hamburger bacteria"), like it, too. In fact, they thrive on it. So all that sugary urine sitting around in your bladder and passing through your ureters and urethra can cause this bacteria to overgrow, resulting in a urinary tract infection (UTI), or cystitis (inflammation of the bladder lining). The longer your urethra is, the more protection you have from UTIs. Men have long urethras; women have very short urethras, however, and in the best of times, are prone to these infections—especially after a lot of sexual activity, which helped to coin the term *honeymoon cystitis*. Sexual intercourse can introduce even more bacteria (from the vagina or rectum) into a woman's urethra due to the close space the vagina and urethra share. Women who wipe from back to front after a bowel movement can also introduce fecal matter into the urethra, causing a UTI.

Any bacterial infection in your bladder area can travel back up to your kidneys, causing infection, inflammation, and a big general mess—again, aggravating all the other problems.

The Smoking Thing

In the same way that smoking contributes to eye complications (see Item 47), it can also aggravate kidney problems. Smoking causes small blood vessel damage throughout your body.

Signs of Diabetes Kidney Disease

Obviously, there are a lot of different problems going on when it comes to diabetes and kidney disease. If you have any of the following early warning signs of kidney disease, see your doctor as soon as possible:

- High blood pressure.
- Protein in the urine (a sign of microvascular problems).
- Burning or difficulty urinating (a sign of a urinary tract infection).
- Foul-smelling or cloudy urine (a sign of a urinary tract infection).
- Pain in the lower abdomen (a sign of a urinary tract infection).
- Blood or pus in the urine (a sign of a kidney infection).
- Fever, chills, or vomiting (a sign of any infection).

- Foamy urine (a sign of kidney infection).
- Frequent urination (a sign of high blood sugar and/or urinary tract infection).

Treating Kidney Disease

If you have high blood pressure, getting it under control through diet, exercise, or blood pressure–lowering medication will help to save your kidneys. If you have high blood sugar, treating any UTI as quickly as possible with antibiotics is the best way to avert kidney infection, while drugs known as ACE inhibitors can help to control small blood vessel damage caused by microvascular complications.

If you wind up with kidney failure, or end-stage renal disease, dialysis or, in the worst-case scenario, a kidney transplant, are the only ways to treat it. Perhaps someday, cloning technology can be used to clone replacement organs, such as kidneys.

50. Understand the Diabetes Control and Complications Trial

A famous study, known as the Diabetes Control and Complications Trial (DCCT) involved 1,441 people with Type 1 diabetes, who were randomly managed according to one of two treatment philosophies: intensive treatment and conventional treatment. Intensive treatment means frequently testing your blood sugar and using a short-acting insulin that requires three to four injections daily, or one dose of longer acting insulin. The goal of this type of management is to achieve blood sugar levels that are as normal as possible as often as possible. Conventional treatment means controlling your diabetes to the point where you avoid feeling any symptoms of high blood sugar, such as frequent urination, thirst, or fatigue, without doing very much, if any, self-testing.

The results of the DCCT were pretty astounding. So much so that the trial, planned for a ten-year period, was cut short—a rare occurrence in research trials. The DCCT results were unveiled in 1993, at the American Diabetes Association's annual conference.

The people who were managed with intensive therapy were able to delay microvascular complications between 35 and 76 percent. Specifically, eye disease was reduced by 76 percent, kidney disease by 56 percent, nerve damage by 61 percent, and high cholesterol by 35 percent. Those are very significant results. Statistically, anything over 1 percent is considered clinically significant. The overwhelming consensus among diabetes practitioners is that intensive therapy for people with Type 1 diabetes prolongs health and greatly reduces complications. Conventional therapy for Type 1 diabetes is now considered archaic and even detrimental.

The National Institute of Diabetes and Digestive and Kidney Diseases (NIDDK) in the United States reported similar findings. NIDDK research found that with intensive therapy, eye disease was reduced by 76 percent, kidney disease by 50 percent, nerve disease by 60 percent, and cardiovascular disease (a macrovascular complication) by 35 percent.

The results of a long-awaited British study on Type 2 diabetes complications were published in 1998. Known as the United Kingdom Prospective Diabetes Study (UKPDS), it set out to determine whether blood sugar control reduces macrovascular complications in Type 2 diabetes, together with lowering blood pressure.

The results show that frequent blood sugar testing can reduce the risk of blindness and kidney failure in people with Type 2 by 25 percent. In those Type 2's with high blood pressure, lowering blood pressure reduced the risk of stroke by 44 percent and of heart failure by 56 percent. And, for every 1 percentage point reduction in the value of the HbA1c test (see Item 4), there was a 35 percent reduction in eye, kidney, and nerve damage and an overall 25 percent reduction in deaths related to diabetes. The bottom line is that the UKPDS shows that frequently self-testing your blood sugar can prevent long-term complications of diabetes for people with Type 2 diabetes, although there was not a direct link between lowering blood sugar and reducing macrovascular complications.

Epilogue

You can live well with Type 2 diabetes, and this book gives you all the tools you need to do that. If you can control your blood sugar (Items 1 through 10), become more active (Items 11 through 20), balance your meals appropriately (Items 21 through 30), and understand how to take your medications and/or insulin properly (Items 31 through 40), you can prevent diabetes complications (Items 41 through 50) and live a full, healthy life.

If you need more information, start by contacting the American Diabetes Association (ADA). (See the resource list.) Plus, every manufacturer of a diabetes product, be it a glucose meter, insulin pen, or diabetes medication, has a toll-free customer care line. These are excellent sources of information. There are also funds made available by several pharmaceutical companies that make various diabetes products to help people with low incomes or insufficient medical coverage to purchase the diabetes care products they need (see Appendix A). In the meantime, if you've found this book helpful, please pass it on to a friend or loved one who may be struggling with managing his or her Type 2 diabetes. Also, visit my website, www.sarahealth.com, for more diabetes information and links.

Appendix A

Drug Money

If you are prescribed any of the following drugs (listed alphabetically), you may be eligible for financial assistance from the drug's manufacturer:

Acarbose

Contact: Bayer Corporation's Indigent Patient Program
1-800-998-9180

Metformin

Contact: Bristol-Myers Squibb's Patient Assistance Program
1-800-437-0994

Insulin (all preparations)

Contact:
Eli Lilly and Company's Lilly Cares Program
1-800-545-6962
Novo Nordisk's Indigent Program
1-800-727-6500

Glyburide or glimepiride

Contact: Hoechst Marion Roussel's Indigent Patient
Program
   1-800-221-4025

Glipizede or chlorpropamide

Contact: Pfizer Prescription Assistance Program
   1-800-646-4455

Note: If you are using other diabetes care products, such
as lancets, glucose meters, and so forth, it's always a good
idea to contact your product manufacturer's customer care
line or toll-free line and ask if assistance programs are
available. These programs are usually not advertised to the
consumer.

Appendix B

Chronology: Diabetes to Date

1552 B.C.E. Earliest known record of diabetes mentioned on Third Dynasty Egyptian papyrus by physician Hesy-Ra; mentions polyuria (frequent urination) as a symptom.

First century A.D.: Diabetes described by Arateus as "the melting down of flesh and limbs into urine."

164 A.D.: Greek physician Galen of Pergamum mistakenly diagnoses diabetes as an ailment of the kidneys.

Prior to eleventh century: Diabetes commonly diagnosed by "water tasters" who drank the urine of people suspected of having diabetes; the urine of people with diabetes was thought to be sweet tasting. *Mellitus*, the Latin word for honey (referring to its sweetness), is added to the term *diabetes* as a result.

1500s: Swiss-born alchemist and physician Paracelsus identifies diabetes as a serious general disorder.

Early 1800s: First chemical tests developed to indicate and measure the presence of sugar in urine.

1800s: French researcher Claude Bernard studies the workings of the pancreas and the glycogen metabolism of the liver.

1800s: Czech researcher I.V. Pavlov discovers the links between the nervous system and gastric secretion, making an important contribution to science's knowledge of the physiology of the digestive system.

Late 1800s: Italian diabetes specialist Catoni isolates his patients under lock and key in order to get them to follow their diets.

Late 1850s: French physician Priorry advises diabetes patients to eat extra-large quantities of sugar as a treatment.

1869: Paul Langerhans, a German medical student, announces in a dissertation that the pancreas contains two systems of cells. One set secretes normal pancreatic juice; the function of the other was unknown. Several years later, these cells are identified as the islets of Langerhans.

1870s: French physician Apollinaire Bouchardat notices the disappearance of glycosuria in his diabetes patients during the rationing of food in Paris while under siege by Germany during the Franco-Prussian War, and formulates the idea of individualized diets for diabetes patients.

1889: Oskar Minkowski and Joseph von Mering at the University of Strasbourg, Austria, first remove the pancreas from a dog to determine the effect of an absent pancreas on digestion. They proved that without its pancreas a dog becomes severely diabetic. They also showed through experiments with duct ligation (surgically tying off different parts of tissue) that the pancreas indeed has two secretions: the external (which feeds directly into the bloodstream and regulates carbohydrate metabolism) and a mysterious internal secretion, which appeared to be the missing secretion in diabetics. This connection between diabetes and the pancreas resulted in a series of early experiments using pancreatic extracts to treat animals and humans. Unfortunately, these experiments didn't work and even served to challenge the entire hypothesis of this internal secretion.

November 14, 1891: Frederick Banting is born near Alliston, Ontario. His parents, devout Methodists, try to pressure their son into joining the ministry; however, Banting instead enrolls in medical school at the University of Toronto in 1912.

February 28, 1899: Charles H. Best is born in West Pembroke, Maine.

1900–1915: Fad diabetes diets include the oat cure (in which the majority of the diet was made up of oatmeal), the milk diet, the rice cure, potato therapy, and even the use of opium.

1906–1907: German scientist Georg Zuelzer makes some interesting progress on June 21, 1906. He injects pancreatic extract under the skin of a comatose fifty-year-old diabetic. The man is momentarily revived, reinforcing the connection between pancreatic extract (pancreatic secretion) and diabetes. Zuelzer obtains funding from the Schering drug company to produce a viable extract for therapy. By 1907, he produces what appears to be a workable pancreatic extract, but Schering decides that the results of his work didn't justify its costs and drops funding. This was unfortunate, considering that Zuelzer's formula was the first pancreatic extract to suppress glycosuria (sugary urine). Zuelzer's extract also caused many toxic side effects, however—what we know today as insulin shock. What should have been a major breakthrough is viewed by pancreatic researchers as a setback. Caution rules, and the risks of these toxic side effects interferes with many pancreatic extract experiments.

1910–1920: Frederick Madison Allen and Elliot P. Joslin emerge as the two leading diabetes specialists in the United States. Joslin believes diabetes to be "the best of the chronic diseases" because it is "clean, seldom unsightly, not contagious, often painless, and susceptible to treatment."

1913: After three years of diabetes study, Frederick Allen publishes *Concerning Glycosuria and Diabetes*, a book that is significant for the revolution in diabetes therapy that developed from it. J. J. R. Macleod, a professor of medicine at the University of Toronto, publishes a book called *Diabetes: Its Pathological Physiology*. Library records show that Frederick Banting borrowed Macleod's book for his research in 1920.

1919: Allen publishes *Total Dietary Regulation in the Treatment of Diabetes*, citing exhaustive case records of 76 of the 100 diabetes patients he observed, and becomes the director of diabetes research at the Rockefeller Institute.

1919–1920: Allen establishes the first treatment clinic in the United States, the Physiatric Institute in New Jersey, to treat patients with diabetes, high blood pressure, and Bright's disease (a kidney disease); wealthy and desperate patients flock to it.

July 1, 1920: Dr. Banting opens his first office in London, Ontario. He receives his first patient on July 29; total earnings for his first month of work are four dollars.

October 30, 1920: Dr. Banting conceives of the idea of insulin after reading Moses Barron's "The Relation of the

Islets of Langerhans to Diabetes with Special Reference to Cases of Pancreatic Lithiasis" in the November issue of *Surgery, Gynecology, and Obstetrics.* In fact, Banting's notebook from that night is fully preserved at the Academy of Medicine in Toronto. In it he writes: "Diabetus. Ligate pancreatic ducts of dogs. Keep dogs alive till acini degenerate leaving Islets. Try to isolate the internal secretion of these to relieve glycosurea."

November 1920: Banting approaches Macleod with his idea. In that meeting, Macleod apparently brings Banting up to date on a variety of research attempts in the area of pancreatic extract. Macleod concedes that no one thought about the fact that the digestive agents of the pancreas may be responsible for destroying the secretion made by the islets of Langerhans. Banting proposes to Macleod that by using duct-ligated pancreases to make an extract, which would destroy the digestive secretions, they could find a treatment for diabetes. (Macleod was apparently irritated by Banting's clear lack of knowledge in the area of diabetes. Nevertheless, it was a good idea! Macleod, it would appear, was sorry the idea never occurred to him.) For the next year, with the assistance of Best, J. B. Collip, and Macleod, Banting continues his research using a variety of different extracts on depancreatized dogs.

December 30, 1921: Banting presents a paper entitled "The Beneficial Influences of Certain Pancreatic Extracts on Pancreatic Diabetes," summarizing his work to this point at a session of the American Physiological Society at Yale University. Among the attendees are Allen and Joslin. Little praise or congratulation is received.

January 23, 1922: One of Banting's insulin extracts is first tested on a human being, a fourteen-year-old boy named

Leonard Thompson, in Toronto; the treatment was considered a success by the end of the following February.

May 21, 1922: James Havens becomes the first American successfully treated with insulin.

May 30, 1922: Pharmaceutical manufacturer Eli Lilly and Company and the University of Toronto collaborate on the mass production of insulin in North America.

October 25, 1923: Banting and Macleod are awarded the Nobel Prize for medicine. Banting shares his award with Best; Macleod then shares his award with Collip. History would not remember Macleod's nor Collip's role in the discovery of insulin. While Banting, Best, Collip, and Macleod would privately acknowledge that they were a team, they could never admit it to each other. For Banting's obituary tribute, Collip wrote that his own contribution to insulin was trivial compared to Banting's. Banting apparently admitted in his later years that he and Best wouldn't have "achieved a damned thing" without Collip.*

---

* In 1978, Banting's first biographer, Lloyd Stevenson, published an article that contained Macleod's personal account of the insulin discovery. Although Macleod had died in 1935, the University of Toronto did not want to reopen old wounds and for many years prevented the publication of that account. Macleod's account was bitter. He left the University of Toronto in 1928 and returned to Scotland as Regius Professor at the University of Aberdeen; it is believed that he moved away from Toronto because he couldn't stand living in the shadow of Banting's idea.

Best replaced Macleod as professor of physiology at the University of Toronto when he was just twenty-nine years old. He went on to enjoy a long, distinguished career, with many awards and honors until he died in 1978. Best continued Macleod's work on the properties of insulin and received delayed credit for insulin's discovery after Banting's death in 1941. The Best Institute was erected next door to the Banting Institute in 1953.

1934: Banting is knighted; he becomes Sir Frederick Banting.

February 21, 1941: Banting is killed in an airplane crash over Newfoundland while en route to England.

1971: Fiftieth anniversary of the discovery of insulin is celebrated worldwide.

1996: Seventy-fifth anniversary of the discovery of insulin is celebrated.**

Collip attempted to invent another version of insulin he called gluclokinin, and then abandoned it. He is also known for pioneering work on parathyroid hormone. Collip received his M.D., and eventually became Chair of Biochemistry at McGill University. He became a world-renowned endocrinologist in Canada, and in 1947 was made Dean of Medicine at the very university that triggered Banting's idea: the University of Western Ontario. Collip enjoyed a great career and died in 1965 at the age of seventy-two.

** New evidence challenges whether Canadians have the right to claim complete ownership of the insulin discovery at all. Romanian scientist Nicolas Paulesco, who was concentrating on measuring the impact of his pancreatic extract (called pancreine) on blood sugar, likely would have been the discoverer of insulin had the Canadians not beaten him to human testing. In 1971, on the fiftieth anniversary of the discovery of insulin, a campaign was launched by Bucharest medical students to honor Paulesco's work and give him due credit.

SOURCES
Bliss, Michael, "Rewriting Medical History," *Journal of History of Medicine and Allied Sciences, Inc.,* 1993, Vol. 48:253–74.
Bliss, Michael, *Banting: A Biography* (Toronto: McClelland & Stewart, 1984.)
Bliss, Michael, *The Discovery of Insulin* (Toronto: McClelland & Stewart, 1982.)
Diabetes Timeline, Canadian Diabetes Association, 1997.
Williams, Michael, J., "J. J. R. Macleod: The Co-Discoverer of Insulin," *Proceedings of the Royal College of Physicians of Edinburgh,* July 1993, Vol. 23, No. 3.

Glossary

Adrenaline: a hormone your body secretes that creates "fight-or-flight" symptoms of increased heart rate, sweating, nervousness, dizziness, and so on.

Aerobic activity: any activity that causes the heart to pump harder and faster, causing you to breathe faster, which increases the level of oxygen in the bloodstream.

Alpha-glucosidase inhibitors (acarbose or Precose): a drug that delays the breakdown of sugar in your meal.

Antihypertension drug: a drug designed to lower blood pressure, sometimes called a "blood thinner."

Biguanides (Metformin): oral hypoglycemic agents that help the body's insulin work better.

Carbohydrates: the building blocks of most foods, which provide energy to the body to fuel the central nervous system; they help the body use vitamins, minerals, amino acids, and other nutrients.

Cholesterol: a whitish, waxy fat made in vast quantities by the liver. (See also HDL; LDL.)

Complex carbohydrates: sophisticated foods that have larger molecules in them, such as grain foods and foods high in fiber.

Creatinine: waste product produced by the muscles and released by the kidneys.

Dextrose tablets: tablets that contain pure dextrose to boost the blood sugar level quickly, in case of hypoglycemia.

Diabetes specialist: an endocrinologist (hormone specialist) who subspecializes in diabetes.

Diabetes: also known as hyperglycemia, which means high blood sugar, a condition in which blood sugar levels are too high; usually defined by a fasting blood sugar level of over 7.8 mmol/L.

Diabetic ketoacidosis (DKA): an emergency situation that can lead to death; signs of DKA include frequent urination, excessive thirst, excessive hunger, and a fruity smell to the breath.

Diabetic neuropathy: diabetic nerve disease; occurs when the cells that comprise nerves are altered in response to high blood sugar.

Diabetic retinopathy: diabetes eye disease, characterized by damage to the back of the eye, or retina.

Diastolic pressure: one of the readings in a blood pressure measurement; the pressure that occurs when the heart rests between contractions.

Fasting blood glucose readings: what your blood sugar levels are before you've eaten.

Fatty acids: crucial nutrients for cells, which also regulate hormone production.

Fiber: part of a plant that cannot be digested, which can lower cholesterol levels or improve regularity; also causes a slower rise in glucose levels, which lowers the body's insulin requirements.

Fructose: a monosaccharide or single sugar that combines with glucose to form sucrose and is one-and-a-half times sweeter than sucrose.

Glucagon: a hormone which, when injected under the skin, causes an increase in blood glucose concentration.

Glucose: a monosaccharide or single sugar that combines with fructose to form sucrose; can also combine with glucose to form maltose, and with galactose to form lactose; slightly less sweet than sucrose.

Glycosylated hemoglobin levels: detailed blood sugar test that checks for glycosylated hemoglobin (glucose attached to the protein in red blood cells), known as glycohemoglobin or HbA1c levels; this test can determine how well blood sugar has been controlled over a period of two to three months by showing what percentage of it is too high.

Guar gum: a good source of fiber made from the seeds of the Indian cluster bean. When you mix guar with water, it turns into a gummy gel, which slows down the digestive system, similar to acarbose.

HDL: high-density lipoproteins, known as the "good cholesterol."

High-fructose corn syrup (HFCS): a liquid mixture of about equal parts glucose and fructose from cornstarch, which has the same sweetness as sucrose.

Human insulin: a type of insulin that is identical to the insulin that is normally produced by the human body.

Hydrogenation: process that converts liquid fat to semi-solid fat by adding hydrogen.

Hyperglycemia: high blood sugar; also known as "diabetes," a condition in which blood sugar levels are too high; defined by a fasting blood sugar level of over 7.8 mmol/L.

Hyperinsulinemia: when the pancreas produces too much insulin; a condition caused by insulin resistance.

Hypertension (high blood pressure): too much tension or force exerted on the artery walls; a condition that damages the small blood vessels as well as the larger arteries.

Hypoglycemia: low blood sugar; defined by a blood sugar level less than 4.0 mmol/L, any time.

Impaired glucose tolerance (IGT): what many doctors refer to as the "gray zone" between normal blood sugar levels and full-blown diabetes.

Insulin Lispro: an insulin analogue (synthetic "copycat") that is very short acting.

Insulin resistance: occurs when the pancreas is making insulin but the cells are not responding to it.

Insulin shock: occurs when low blood sugar is caused by insulin therapy.

Insulin: a hormone made by the islets of Langerhans, a small island of cells afloat in the pancreas, which regulates blood sugar levels.

Intensive insulin therapy: a treatment program involving close monitoring of blood sugar levels combined with taking short-acting insulin prior to meals.

Islets of Langerhans: one of two cell systems located inside the pancreas, which secretes insulin.

Lancet: tiny needle used to prick the finger for a blood sample.

LDL: low-density lipoproteins, known as the "bad cholesterol."

Leptin: A hormone currently being used to treat obesity (leptin deficiency is thought to contribute to obesity).

Macrovascular complication: a large blood vessel complication, one that is bodywide, or systemic, such as cardiovascular problems.

Microvascular complication: a problem with the smaller blood vessels (capillaries) that connect to various body parts, such as the eyes.

Nonnutritive sweeteners: sugar substitutes or artificial sweeteners, such as saccharin and sucralose, that do not have any calories and will not affect blood sugar levels.

Nutritive sweeteners: sweeteners such as table sugar, molasses, and honey, which have calories or contain natural sugar.

Obesity: when you weigh more than 20 percent over your ideal weight for your age and height.

Omega-3 fatty acids: substances naturally present in fish that swim in cold waters; crucial for brain tissue, are all polyunsaturated, and not only lower cholesterol levels, but protect against heart disease.

Oral glucose tolerance test: Standard method of diagnosing impaired glucose tolerance (IGT) or diabetes; blood sugar is tested every thirty minutes for two hours following a period of fasting.

Oral hypoglycemic agents (OHAs): drugs that help the pancreas release more insulin or help insulin work more effectively.

Orlistat: an antiobesity drug that blocks the absorption of almost one-third of the fat one consumes.

Pancreas: a birdbeak–shaped gland situated behind the stomach.

Peripheral vascular disease (PVD): occurs when blood flow to the limbs (arms, legs, and feet) is blocked, causing cramping, pains, or numbness.

Premixed insulin: when both short-acting insulin and intermediate-acting insulin are mixed together.

Renin: a hormone produced by the kidneys which helps to regulate blood pressure.

Saturated fat: a fat that is solid at room temperature (from animal sources) that stimulates the body to produce LDL, or "bad cholesterol."

Soluble fiber: fiber that is water soluble, or dissolves in water; it forms a gel in the body that traps fats and lowers cholesterol.

Stroke: occurs when a blood clot travels to the brain and stops the flow of blood and oxygen carried to the nerve cells in that area, at which point cells may die or vital body functions controlled by the brain may be temporarily or permanently damaged.

Sucrose: A disaccharide, or double sugar made of equal parts glucose and fructose; known as table or white sugar; found naturally in sugar cane and sugar beets.

Sugar alcohols: nutritive sweeteners that are half as sweet as sugar; found naturally in fruits or manufactured from carbohydrates (sorbitol).

Sulphonylureas: oral hypoglycemic agents that help the pancreas release more insulin.

Systolic pressure: one of the readings in a blood pressure measurement; the pressure that occurs during the heart's contraction.

Thiazoladinediones (troglitazone or Rezulin): agents that make the cells more sensitive to insulin.

Trans-fatty acids (hydrogenated oils): harmful, man-made fats that not only raise the level of "bad cholesterol" (LDL) in the bloodstream, but lower the amount of "good cholesterol" (HDL) that's already there; produced through the process of hydrogenation.

Triglycerides: a combination of saturated, monounsaturated, and polyunsaturated fatty acids and glycerol.

Type 1 diabetes: insulin-dependent diabetes mellitus (IDDM), a disease usually diagnosed before age thirty, in which the pancreas stops producing insulin; Type 1 diabetes, also known as juvenile diabetes, requires daily insulin injections for life.

Type 2 diabetes: non-insulin-dependent diabetes mellitus (NIDDM), also called late-onset or mature-onset diabetes because it's usually diagnosed after age forty-five; the body either does not produce enough insulin or the insulin it does produce cannot be used efficiently.

Unsaturated fat: known as "good fat" because it doesn't cause the body to produce "bad cholesterol" and increases the levels of "good cholesterol;" partially solid or liquid at room temperature.

Urea: the waste product of protein released by the kidneys.

Where to Go for More Information

Note: This list was compiled from dozens of sources. Because of the nature of many health and nonprofit organizations, some of the addresses and phone numbers may have changed since this list was compiled. Many of these organizations have e-mail addresses, some of which are not made public. Please review sarahealth.com links at the end of this list.

American Association of Diabetes Educators
    500 N. Michigan Avenue, Suite 1400
    Chicago, IL 60611
    1-800-388-DMED or (312) 661-1700
    http://www.aadenet.org/

The American Diabetes Association
    ADA National Service Center
    1660 Duke Street
    Alexandria, VA 22314
    1-800-232-6733 or (703) 549-1500

American Foundation for the Blind
    11 Penn Plaza, Suite 300
    New York, NY 10001
    (212) 502-7661; fax (212) 502-7777

American Heart Association
    7320 Greenville Pike
    Dallas, TX 75231
    (214) 373-6300

American National Kidney Foundation
    30 East 33rd Street
    New York, NY 10016
    1-800-622-9010 or (212) 889-2210

Canadian Diabetes Association
    15 Toronto Street, Suite 800
    Toronto, ON M5C 2E3
    (416) 363-3373; fax (416) 363-3393
    http://www.diabetes.ca

Diabetes Research and Wellness Foundation
    (provides free medical alert ID necklaces and
    diabetes self-management diaries)
    P.O. Box 3837
    Merrifield, VA 22116
    (202) 298-9211
    http://www.charities.org/dirs/health/drwf/index.html

International Diabetes Center
    3800 Park Nicollet Boulevard
    St. Louis Park, MN 55416
    (612) 993-3393

International Diabetes Federation
    International Association Center
    40 Washington Street
    B-1050 Brussels, Belgium
    32-2-647-4414
    http://www.idf.org/

International Diabetic Athletes Association
    1647-B West Bethany Home Road
    Phoenix, AZ 85015
    (602) 433-2113

Joslin Diabetes Center
    1 Joslin Place
    Boston, MA 02215
    (617) 732-2415
    http://www.joslin.org/

MedicAlert Foundation
    2323 Colorado Avenue
    Turlock, CA 95382
    1-800-825-3785

National Diabetes Information Clearinghouse
    Box NDIC
    Bethesda, MD 20892
    (301) 468-2162

National Diabetes Outreach Program
    One Diabetes Way
    Bethesda, MD 20892-3600
    1-800-438-5383

National Federation of the Blind
    1800 Johnston Street
    Baltimore, MD 21230
    (410) 659-9314
    http://www.nfb.org

National Osteoporosis Foundation
    1150 17th Street NW, Suite 500
    Washington, DC 20036-4603
    1-800-223-9994 or (202) 223-2226

Food/Nutrition

American Anorexia/Bulimia Association, Inc.
    133 Cedar Lane
    Teaneck, NJ 07666
    (201) 836-1800

Anorexia Nervosa and Related Eating Disorders, Inc.
    P.O. Box 5102
    Eugene, OR 97405
    (503) 344-1144

Bulimia, Anorexia Self-Help (BASH)
    6125 Clayton Avenue, Suite 215
    St. Louis, MO 63139
    1-800-BASH-STL or (314) 991-BASH

National Anorexic Aid Society
    5796 Karl Road
    Columbus, Ohio 43229
    (614) 436-1112

Grocery Manufacturers of America
    1010 Wisconsin Avenue NW, Suite 900
    Washington, DC 20007
    (202) 337-9400; fax (202) 337-4508

National Food Safety Database
U.S. Department of Agriculture
Dr. Mark Tamplin
University of Florida
Old Dairy Science, Building 120, Room 105
Box 110365
Gainesville, FL 32611-0365
E-mail: mlt@gnv.ifas.ufl.edu

Organic Trade Association
50 Miles Street
P.O. Box 1078
Greenfield, MA 01302
(413) 774-7511
E-mail: ota@igc.apc.org

Overeaters Anonymous
P.O. Box 44020
Rio Rancho, NM 87174-4402
(505) 891-2664

Toll-Free Hotlines

American Dietetic Association and National Center for
Nutrition and Dietetics (NCND) Consumer Nutrition
1-800-366-1655

American Podiatric Medical Association
1-800-FOOTCARE

Pharmaceutical Company Customer Care Lines

Bayer Diagnostics Division
1-800-348-8100

Boehringer Mannheim Corporation
1-800-858-8072

LifeScan, a Johnson & Johnson Company
    1-800-227-8862

MediSense, Inc.
    1-800-527-3339

Novo Nordisk Pharmaceuticals
    1-800-727-6500

Cascade Medical
    1-800-525-6718

Links from sarahealth.com

For more information about disease prevention and wellness, visit me online at www.sarahealth.com, where you will find over three hundred links—including these—related to your good health and wellness.

- American Diabetes Association.
  www.diabetes.org
- Canadian Diabetes Association.
  www.diabetes.ca
- American Association of Clinical Endocrinologists.
  www.aace.com
- National Institute of Diabetes and Digestive Kidney Disease.
  www.niddk.nih.gov/
- Amputation Prevention Global Resource Center: prevention, causes, signs and symptoms, treatment.
  www.diabetesresource.com

- About.com (Diabetes).
  http://diabetes.about.com.health/diabetes/mbody.htm

- Diabetes mall: targets both a general audience and medical professionals. Information about research, prevention, and education. With support group.
  www.diabetesnet.com/index.html

- Diabetes monitor: great source of patient information, research, statistics, and education. Registry of links.
  www.diabetesmonitor.com

- National Diabetes Fact Sheet (from the U.S. Centers for Disease Control and Prevention).
  www.cdc.gov/diabetes

- National Diabetes Information Clearinghouse (and diabetes database).
  www.niddk.nih.gov/NDIC/NDIC.html

- NutraSweet: facts about this artificial sugar substitute.
  www.alaskanet:/80/~tne/

- Olestra: information about this synthetic fat product now available in the United States.
  www.diabetesmonitor.com/olestra.htm

- Recipe of the Day: features a new healthy recipe every day, Monday through Thursday. From the ADA.
  www.diabetes.org/ada/rcptoday.html

- Managing Your Diabetes: official site of Eli Lilly and Company. Lots of great information about diabetes products.
  http://diabetes.lilly.com

- Blindness and Diabetes Resource and Support: includes back issues of the *Voice of the Diabetic* from the National Federation of the Blind.
  www.prevent-blindness.org

- MedicAlert: site of the trademarked MedicAlert emblem.
  www.medicalert.org

- Diabetes Type 2 Resource and Discussion Page: information specific to those with Type 2 Diabetes.
  http://home.ptd.net/~hwagner/2r.htm

- Diabetes Type 2: from the American Medical Association; symptoms, screening, diagnosis, complications, and so on.
  www.ama-assn.org/insight/spe_con/diabetes.htm

- Diabetes.com (Diabetes and Sexual Intimacy): award-winning site with health library, products, and prescriptions, newsroom.
  www.diabetes.com/site/

- Diabetic Gourmet Magazine: free newsletter, daily tidbits, menus, and forum.
  http://gourmetconnection.com/diabetic/

- HealthNet—Diabetes: treatment, patient education, advice.
  www.healthnet.com

- The Islet Foundation: foundation dedicated to finding a cure for insulin-dependent diabetes. Interesting resources and information on the future of diabetes.
  www.islet.org

Diabetes Glucose Meters

- The Roche Group (Accu-Check).
  www.roche.com

- Polymer Tech Systems, Inc.
  www.diabetes-testing.com

- LXN Corp.
  www.lxncorp.com

- LifeScan, Inc.
  United States—www.lifescan.com
  Canada—www.lifescan-can.com

- Chronimed, Inc.
  www.chronimed.com

- QuestStar Medical, Inc.
  www.queststarmedical.com

- Bayer Corp.
  www.glucometer.com/product.htm

- Abbott Laboratories.
  www.abbott.com

Bibliography

Abbott Hommel Cynthia, "The SUGAR group." *Diabetes Dialogue* (Vol. 41, No. 3), Fall 1994.

"Acarbose (Prandase)." *New Drugs/Drug News*, Ontario College of Pharmacists Drug Information Service Newsletter (Vol. 14, No. 2), March/April 1996.

Accu-Chek Advantage System, The. Patient information, Eli Lilly of Canada, Inc., distributed 1997.

"Advocacy in action." *Diabetes Dialogue* (Vol. 43, No. 3), Fall 1996.

"Agony of de-feet, The." *Equilibrium*, Canadian Diabetes Association (No. 1), 1996.

Alcohol and Diabetes—Do They Mix? Booklet, Canadian Diabetes Association, 1996.

All About Insulin. Booklet, Novo Nordisk Canada, Inc., 1996.

All About Insulin: Novolin Care. Patient information manual, Novo Nordisk Canada, Inc.

Allard, Johane P., MD, FRCP. Excerpts from "International conference on antioxidant vitamins and beta-carotene in disease prevention: A Canadian perspective." 1996.

Allsop, Karen F., and Janette Brand Miller. "Honey revisited: A reappraisal of honey in preindustrial diets." *British Journal of Nutrition* (Vol. 75)1996:513–20.

American Diabetes Association. "An introduction to oral medications for diabetes." Posted to Diabetes.com, January 1999.

———. "Carbohydrate counting: A new way to plan meals." Posted to Diabetes.com, January 1999.

———. "Standards of medical care for patients with diabetes mellitus." *Diabetes Care* (Vol. 21, Supplement 1), *Clinical Practice Recommendations 1998.*

———. "The United Kingdom Prospective Diabetes Study (UKPDS) for Type 2 diabetes: What you need to know about the results of a long-term study." Posted to: www.diabetes.org, January 1999.

———. Online information. Document ID: ADA035, 1995.

Anderson, Pauline. "Researchers predict 'beginning of the end' of diabetes." *The Medical Post*, August 22, 1995.

Antioxidant Connection: Visiting Speakers Discuss Immunity, Diabetes, The. Vitamin Information Program, Hoffman-La Roche, Ltd., September 1995.

Antonucci, T., et al. "Impaired glucose tolerance is normalized by treatment with the thiazoladinedione. *Diabetes Care* (Vol. 20, No. 2), February 1997:188–93.

Appavoo, Donna, Rayanne Waboose, and Stuart Harris. "Sioux lookout diabetes program." *Diabetes Dialogue* (Vol. 41, No. 3), Fall 1994.

Armstrong, David G., Lawrence A. Lavery, and Lawrence B. Harkless. "Treatment-based classification system for assessment and care of diabetic feet." *Journal of the American Podiatric Medical Association* (Vol. 87, No. 7), July 1996.

Badley, Wendy. "Across the country." *Diabetes Dialogue* (Vol. 41, No. 3), Fall 1994.

Balancing Your Blood Sugar: A Guide for People with Diabetes. Patient information from Canadian Diabetes Association, distributed 1997.

"Bayer launches major international research project into prevention of diabetes." Media Release, March 5, 1997.

Berndl, Leslie. "Understanding fat." *Diabetes Dialogue* (Vol. 42, No.1), Spring 1995.

Better Health & Medical Network Collective Work & Database. Transmitted to the Internet, August 18, 1997.

Beyers, Joanne. "How sweet it is!" *Diabetes Dialogue* (Vol. 42, No.1), Spring 1995.

Biermann, June, and Barbara Toohey. *The Diabetic's Book.* (New York: Perigee Books, 1992).

Blood Glucose Monitoring: Guidelines to a Healthier You. Patient information from Bayer, Inc., Healthcare division, distributed 1997.

Blood Pressure: Check It Out. Countdown USA: Countdown to a Healthy Heart, Allegheny General Hospital and Voluntary Hospitals of America, Inc., 1990.

Blood Sugar Testing Diary. Patient information, Becton Dickinson Consumer Products, 1996.

Bonen, Arent. "Fueling your tank." *Diabetes Dialogue* (Vol. 42, No. 4), Winter 1995.

Bril, Vera. "Diabetic neuropathy: Can it be treated?" *Diabetes Dialogue* (Vol. 41, No. 4), Winter 1994.

Brubaker, Patricia L. "Glucagon-like peptide-1." *Diabetes Dialogue* (Vol. 41, No. 4), Winter 1994.

Canadian Diabetes Association. "Health . . . the smoke-free way." *Equilibrium* (No. 1), 1996.

Canadian Medical Association Journal and the Canadian Diabetes Association. "1998 clinical practice guidelines for the management of diabetes in Canada." Supplement to *Canadian Medical Association Journal* (8 Suppl), 1998:159.

Cattral, Mark. "Pancreas transplantation." *Diabetes Dialogue* (Vol. 43, No. 4), Winter 1996.

Chaddock, Brenda. "Activity is key to diabetes health." *Canadian Pharmacy Journal*, March 1997.

———. "Foul weather fitness: The hardest part is getting started." *Canadian Pharmacy Journal*, March 1996.

———. "The magic of exercise." *Canadian Pharmacy Journal*, September 1995.

———. "The right way to read a label." *Canadian Pharmacy Journal*, May 1996.

———. "Blood-glucose testing: Keep up with the trend." *Canadian Pharmacy Journal*, September 1996:17.

———. "Doing the things that make a difference." *Canadian Pharmacy Journal*, July/August 1996.

Challenge: Newsletter of the International Diabetic Athletes Association, The. (Vol. 11, No. I), Spring 1997.

Choosing Your Sweetener. Product information, PROSWEET Canada, 1997.

Christrup, Janet. "Nuts about nuts: The joys of growing nut trees." *Cognition*, July 1991:20–22.

Clarke, Bill. "Action Figures." *Diabetes Dialogue* (Vol. 43, No. 3), Fall 1996.

Clarke, Peter V. "Hemoglobin A1c test helps long-term diabetes management." *Monitor* (Vol. 1, No. 1), MediSense Canada, Inc.

"Complications: The long-term picture." *Equilibrium*, Canadian Diabetes Association (No. 1), 1996.

Cronier, Claire. "Sweetest choices." *Diabetes Dialogue* (Vol. 44, No. 1), Spring 1997.

Dextrolog: for Recording Blood and Urine Glucose Test Results. Booklet, Bayer, Inc., Healthcare Division, distributed 1997.

Diabetes and Kidney Disease. Patient information, the Kidney Foundation of Canada, 1995.

Diabetes and Nonprescription Drugs: Guidelines to a Healthier You. Patient information, Bayer, Inc., Healthcare Division, distributed 1997.

"Diabetes: An undetected time-bomb." *CARP News*, April 1996.

"Diabetes: Facts and figures." *News from the VIP* (No. 2), Fall 1995. Vitamin Information Program, Fine Chemicals Division of Hoffman-La Roche, Ltd.

"Diabetes implants tested." *Los Angeles Daily News*, January 23, 1997.

"Diabetes: What is it?" *Equilibrium*, Canadian Diabetes Association (No. 1), 1996.

"Diets slow reaction times." *Reuters*, April 8, 1997.

"Discovery of insulin marked turning point in human history." *The Globe and Mail*, November 1, 1996.

"*Double Trouble*." Countdown USA: Countdown to a Healthy Heart, Allegheny General Hospital and Voluntary Hospitals of America, Inc., 1990.

Doyle, Patricia. *Insulin — The Facts*. Canadian Diabetes Association, 1995.

Drum, David, and Terry Zierenberg. *The Type 2 Diabetes Sourcebook* (Los Angeles: Lowell House, 1998).

Dutcher, Lisa. "A wholistic approach to diabetes management." *Diabetes Dialogue* (Vol. 41, No. 3), Fall 1994.

Engel, June V. "Beyond vitamins: Phytochemicals to help fight disease." *University of Toronto Health News* (Vol. 14), June 1996.

———. "Eating fiber." *Diabetes Dialogue* (Vol. 44, No. 1), Spring 1997.

Exercise: Guidelines to a Healthier You. Patient information, Bayer, Inc., Healthcare Division, distributed 1997.

Expert Committee on the Diagnosis and Classification of Diabetes Mellitus, Report of the Expert Committee on the Diagnosis and Classification of Diabetes Mellitus, The. American Diabetes Association, January 1, 1998.

Farquhar, Andrew. "Exercising essentials." *Diabetes Dialogue* (Vol. 43, No. 3), Fall 1996:6–8.

Fat Trap, Countdown USA: Countdown to a Healthy Heart, The.
Allegheny General Hospital and Voluntary Hospitals
of America, Inc., 1990.

"FDA approves drug to reduce insulin needs for some
diabetics." The Associated Press, January 30, 1997.

"First New Insulin in 14 Years Approved for Use in
Canada." Media Release, Eli Lilly of Canada,
Inc./Boehringer Mannheim Canada, October 9, 1996.

"Following the patient with chronic disease." *Patient Care
Canada* (Vol. 7, No. 5), May 1996:22–38.

"Following the patient with stable chronic disease: Type II
diabetes mellitus." *Patient Care Canada* (Vol. 7, No. 5),
May 1996.

Food and Drug Administration. "Nutrient claims guide for
individual foods." *Special Report, Focus on Food Labeling,*
FDA Publication no. 95-2289.

Food and Exercise: Guidelines to a Healthier You. Patient
information, Bayer, Inc., Healthcare Division,
distributed 1997.

Fraser, Elizabeth, and Bill Clarke. "Loafing around."
Diabetes Dialogue (Vol. 44, No.1), Spring 1997.

Gabrys, Jennifer. "Ask the professionals." *Diabetes Dialogue*
(Vol. 43, No. 4), Winter 1996.

Gauthier, Serge G., and Patricia H. Coleman. "Nutrition
and aging." *The Lederle Letter* (Vol. 2, No. 2), April
1993.

Glucometer Elite. Patient information, Bayer Healthcare
Division, 1995.

Gordon, Dennis. "Acarbose: When it works/when it
doesn't." *Diabetes Forecast*, February 1997.

Guthrie, Diana, and Richard A. Guthrie. *The Diabetes Sourcebook* (Los Angeles: Lowell House, 1996).

Harrison, Pam. "Rethinking obesity." *Family Practice*, March 11, 1996.

Health Record for People with Diabetes. Patient information booklet, Canadian Diabetes Association/LifeScan Canada, Ltd, McNeil Consumer Products Company, 1996.

Heart Healthy Kitchen, The. Countdown USA: Countdown to a Healthy Heart, Allegheny General Hospital and Voluntary Hospitals of America, Inc., 1990.

Heart Disease and Stroke. Patient information, Heart and Stroke Foundation of Ontario, distributed 1997.

High Blood Pressure and Your Kidneys. Patient information, Kidney Foundation of Canada, 1995.

"High-carbohydrate diet not for everyone." *Reuters*, April 16, 1997.

Ho, Marian. "Learning your ABCs, part two." *Diabetes Dialogue* (Vol. 43, No. 3), Fall 1996.

"Hostility and heart risk." *Reuters Health Summary*, April 22, 1997.

Houlden, Robyn. "Health beliefs in two Ontario First Nations populations." *Diabetes Dialogue* (Vol. 41, No. 4), Winter 1994.

"How adults are learning to manage diabetes with their lifestyle." *The Globe and Mail*, November 1, 1996.

How Do I Choose a Healthy Diet? Patient information, Heart and Stroke Foundation of Ontario, distributed 1997.

How to Choose Your New Blood Glucose Meter. Patient information, LifeScan Canada, Inc., distributed 1997.

How to Cope with a Brief Illness: A Guide for the Person Taking Insulin. Patient information, the Canadian Diabetes Association, March 1996.

How to Take Insulin. Patient information, Monoject Diabetes Care Products, distributed 1997.

Hunt, John A. "Fueling up." *Diabetes Dialogue* (Vol. 41, No. 4), Winter 1994.

Hunter, J. E., and T. H. Applewhite. "Reassessment of trans-fatty acid availability in the U.S. diet." *American Journal of Clinical Nutrition* (Vol. 54), 1991:363–69.

Hurley, Jane, and Stephen Schmidt. "Going with the grain." *Nutrition Action*, October 1994:10–11.

IFIC Review: Intense Sweeteners: Effects on Appetite and Weight Management. International Food Information Council, Washington, D.C., November 1995.

IFIC Review: Uses and Nutritional Impact of Fat Reduction Ingredients. International Food Information Council, Washington, D.C., October 1995.

"Improving treatment outcomes in NIDDM: The questions and controversies." *Diabetes Report* (Vol. 2, No. 1), 1996.

"Insulin and Type 2 diabetes." *Equilibrium*, Canadian Diabetes Association (No. 1), 1996.

Insulin: Guidelines to a Healthier You. Patient information, Bayer, Inc., Healthcare Division, distributed 1997.

Insulin Management Information. Patient information, Eli Lilly and Co., distributed 1997.

Is Your Insulin as Easy to Use as Humulin? Patient information, Eli Lilly of Canada, Inc., distributed 1997.

Jovanovic-Peterson, Lois, June Biermann, and Barbara Toohey. *The Diabetic Woman: All Your Questions Answered* (New York: G.P. Putnam's Sons, 1996.)

Joyce, Carol. "What's new in Type 2." *Diabetes Dialogue* (Vol. 43, No. 3), Fall 1996.

Keeping Well with Diabetes: Novolin Care. Patient information, Novo Nordisk Canada, Inc., 1996.

Kermode-Scott, Barbara. "NIDDM affecting huge numbers, says expert." *Family Practice*, March 11, 1996.

Kidney Stones. Patient information, Kidney Foundation of Canada, 1995.

Korytkowski, Mary. "Something old, something new." *Diabetes Spectrum* (Vol. 9, No. 4), November 1996.

Kuczmarski, R.J., K.M. Flegal, S.M. Campbell, and C.L. Johnson. "Increasing prevalence of overweight among U.S. adults: The national health and nutrition examination surveys, 1960 to 1991." *Journal of the American Medical Association* (Vol. 272), 1994:205–11.

Kumar, S., et al. "Troglitazone, an insulin action enhancer, improves metabolic control in NIDDM patients." *Diabetologia* (Vol. 30, No. 6), June 1996:701–9.

Lebovitz, Harold E. "Acarbose, an alpha-glucosidase inhibitor, in the treatment of NIDDM." *Diabetes Care* (Vol. 19, Suppl. 1), 1996:554–61.

Leiter, Lawrence A. "Acarbose: New treatment in NIDDM patients, new drugs/drug news." *Ontario College of Pharmacists* (Vol. 14, No. 2).

Lichtenstein, A. H., et al. "Hydrogenation impairs the hypolipidemic effect of corn oil in humans." *Arteriosclerosis and Thrombosis* (Vol. 13), 1993:154–61.

Linden, Ron. "Hyperbaric medicine." *Diabetes Dialogue* (Vol. 43, No. 4), Fall 1996.

Little, Linda. "Vitamin E may help cut diabetics' risk of heart disease." *Medical Post*, May 14, 1996:5.

Little, Margaret. "Step right up." *Diabetes Dialogue* (Vol. 43, No. 3), Fall 1996.

Living Well. Patient information, Canadian Diabetes Association, distributed 1997.

"Low blood Sugars: Your questions answered." *Equilibrium*, Canadian Diabetes Association (No. 1), 1996.

MacMillan, Harriet L., Angus B. MacMillan, David R. Offord, and Jennifer L. Dingle. "Aboriginal health." *Canadian Medical Association Journal* (Vol. 155), 1996:1569–78.

Managing Your Diabetes with Humalog. Booklet, Eli Lilly and Company, 1997.

Marliss, Errol B., and Rejeanne Gougeon. "Focus on women: Dieting as a possible risk factor for obesity." *The Lederle Letter* (Vol. 2, No. 4), August 1993.

Marliss, Errol B., Rejeanne Gougeon, and Sandra Schwenger. "Weight-reducing diets may compromise nutrition." *The Lederle Letter* (Vol. 1, No. 3), August 1992.

Martin, Cheryl. "Acarbose (Prandase)." *Communication*, March/April 1996:38.

Mature Lifestyles: High Blood Pressure. Patient information, Health Watch/Shoppers Drug Mart, distributed 1997.

MediSense Blood Glucose Sensor. Product mongraph, 1995.

Micral-S Kidney Chek. Patient information, Eli Lilly of Canada/Boehringer Mannheim Canada, Inc., distributed 1997.

"Monitoring your blood sugar." *Equilibrium*, Canadian Diabetes Association (No. 1), 1996.

Monoject: Diabetes Care Products. Patient information, Sherwood Medical Industries Canada, Inc., distributed 1997.

Musgrove, Lorraine. "Ask the professionals." *Diabetes Dialogue* (Vol. 44, No. 1), Spring 1997:60–61.

Neergaard, Lauran. "Study finds low hormone levels may encourage weight gain." Associated Press, May 14, 1997.

Neuschwander-Tetri, B.A., et al. "Troglitazone-induced hepatic failure leading to liver transplantation: A case report." *Annals of Internal Medicine* (Vol. 129), July 1, 1998:38–41.

"New developments in the management of Type II diabetes." *Diabetes Report* (Vol. 1, No. 2), 1995.

"New perspectives in the management of NIDDM." *Diabetes Report* (Vol. 1, No. 3), 1996.

Non-Insulin Dependent Diabetes Mellitus. Patient information, National Pharmacy Continuing Education Program and Bayer, Inc., February 1997.

Novolin ge: Insulin, Human Biosynthetic Antidiabetic Agent. Product Monograph for Novo Nordisk Canada, Inc., 1997.

Nutrition for Diabetes. Patient information, Novo Nordisk Canada, Inc., 1996.

"Nutrition news." *Diabetes Dialogue* (Vol. 43, No. 4), Winter 1996.

"Nutrition news." *Diabetes Dialogue* (Vol. 44, No.1), Spring 1997.

"Nutrition principles for the management of diabetes and related complications." *Diabetes Care* (Vol. 17), 1994:490–518.

"Oats are in." *Countdown USA: Countdown to a Healthy Heart*, Allegheny General Hospital and Voluntary Hospitals of America, Inc., 1990.

"Olestra: yes or no?" *University of California at Berkeley Wellness Letter*, in *Diabetes Dialogue* (Vol. 43, No. 3), Fall 1996.

One Touch Profile: For Complete Diabetes Management. Patient information, LifeScan Canada, Inc., distributed 1997.

"Physical activity." *Equilibrium*, Canadian Diabetes Association (No. 1), 1996.

"Pills for diabetes?" *Equilibrium*, Canadian Diabetes Association (No. 1), 1996.

"Pills for treating diabetes." Patient information, Canadian Diabetes Association, March 1996.

Pocket Partner: A Guide to Healthy Food Choices. Booklet, Canadian Diabetes Association, distributed 1997.

Pocket Serving Sizer. Patient information, Canadian Diabetes Association, distributed 1997.

Poirier, Laurinda M., and Katharine M. Coburn. *Women & Diabetes: Life Planning for Health and Wellness* (New York: Bantam Books, 1997).

"Position of the American Dietetic Association: Use of nutritive and nonnutritive sweeteners." *Journal of the American Dietetic Association* (Vol. 93), 1993:816–22.

Practical Advice for the Prandase Patient. Booklet, Bayer, Inc., Healthcare Division, distributed 1996.

Prandase (Acarbose) Tablets. Product monograph, Bayer, Inc., Healthcare Division, April 14, 1997.

Prandase: A New Approach to NIDDM Therapy. Patient information booklet, Bayer, Inc., Healthcare Division, distributed 1997.

Preventing the Complications of Diabetes: Guidelines to a Healthier You. Patient information, Bayer, Inc., Healthcare Division, distributed 1997.

"Prevention and treatment of obesity: application to Type 2 diabetes." *Diabetes Care* (Vol. 20), 1997:1744–66.

Prochaska, James O. "A revolution in diabetes evaluation." Canadian Diabetes Association Conference, 1995.

"Proper knowledge of a healthy diet makes huge difference." *The Globe and Mail*, November 1, 1996.

PROSWEET: The Low-Calorie Pure Sugar Taste Sweetener. Product information, PROSWEET Canada, 1997.

"Protein content of the diabetic diet." *Diabetes Care* (Vol. 17), 1994:1502–13.

Putting Fun Back into Food. International Food Information Council, Washington, D.C., 1997.

"Q & A about fatty acids and dietary fats." International Food Information Council, Washington, D.C., 1997.

"Q & A on low-calorie sweeteners." *Diabetes News* (Vol. 1, No. 2), Spring 1997.

Real-World Factors That Interfere with Blood-Glucose Meter Accuracy. Patient information, MediSense Canada, Inc., 1996.

"Receptor, The." *Canadian Association for Familial Hypercholesterolemia* (Vol. 7, No. 3), Fall/Winter 1996.

Reddy, Sethu. "Smoking and diabetes." *Diabetes Dialogue* (Vol. 42, No. 4), Winter 1995.

Reducing Your Risk of Diabetes Complications. Patient information, MediSense Canada, Inc., distributed 1997.

Report on the Second International Conference on Diabetes and Native Peoples. First Nations Health Commission, Assembly of First Nations, November 1993.

"Research, improvement in products never stops in health industry." *The Globe and Mail*, November 1, 1996.

Rosenthal, M. Sara. *Managing Your Diabetes* (Toronto: Macmillan Canada, 1997).

―――. *The Type 2 Diabetic Woman* (Chicago: NTC/Contemporary, 1999).

Ruggiero, Laura. *Helping People with Diabetes Change: Practical Applications of the Stages of Change Model.* Professional information, LifeScan Education Institute, distributed 1997.

Ryan, David. "At the controls." *Diabetes Dialogue* (Vol. 43, No. 3), Fall 1996.

Schoepp, Glen. "What is the role of acarbose (Prandase) in diabetes management?" *Pharmacy Practice* (Vol. 12, No. 4), April 1996:37–38.

Schwartz, Carol. "An eye-opener." *Diabetes Dialogue* (Vol. 43, No. 4), Winter 1996.

Seto, Carol. "Nutrition labeling—U.S. style." *Diabetes Dialogue*, Canadian Diabetes Association (Vol. 42, No.1), Spring 1995.

7 Key Factors for Real World Accuracy in the Real World. Patient information, MediSense Canada, Inc., distributed 1997.

7 Key Steps to Control Your Diabetes. Patient information from MediSense Canada, Inc., distributed 1997.

"Seven tips for your sick day blues." *Equilibrium*, Canadian Diabetes Association (No. 1), 1996.

Sinclair, A.J. "Rational approaches to the treatment of patients with non-insulin-dependent diabetes mellitus." *Practical Diabetes Supplement* (Vol. 10, No. 6), November/December 1993.

Sorting Out the Facts About Fat. International Food Information Council, Washington, D.C., 1997.

"Spring at last!" *Diabetes News*, LifeScan Education Institute, Spring 1996.

Stehlin, Dori. "A Little Lite Reading." Posted to FDA website: http://www.fda.gov/fdac/foodlabel/diabetes.html.

Sucralose Overview. Product information, Splenda Information Center, 1997.

Surestep. Patient information, LifeScan Canada, Inc., distributed 1997.

"Sweet promise from sugar substitute?" *Medical Post*, July 2, 1996.

Taking Care of Your Feet: Guidelines to a Healthier You. Patient information, Bayer, Inc., Healthcare Division, distributed 1997.

10 Tips to Healthy Eating. American Dietetic Association and National Center for Nutrition and Dietetics (NCND), April 1994.

Todd, Robert. "The sporting life." *Diabetes Dialogue* (Vol. 43, No. 4), Fall 1996.

Traveling with Diabetes. Patient information, Canadian Diabetes Association, March 1996.

Treating Kidney Failure. Patient information, Kidney Foundation of Canada, 1995.

Type II Diabetes. Shoppers Drug Mart Education Series NIDDM (Vol. 95):11.

Understanding Type 2 Diabetes: Guidelines for a Healthier You. Patient information, Bayer, Inc., Healthcare Division, distributed 1997.

Wanless, Melanie. "The weight debate." *Diabetes Dialogue* (Vol. 44, No. 1), Spring 1997.

Watch Your Step. Booklet, Novo Nordisk Canada, Inc., 1996.

We're Winning: By Changing Lifestyles, We're Proving Every Day That Coronary Disease Can Be Beaten, Countdown USA: Countdown to a Healthy Heart, Allegheny General Hospital and Voluntary Hospitals of America, Inc., 1990.

What Is Diabetes? Canadian Diabetes Association, February 2, 1996. CDA Document ID: ADA037.

What Is Intensive Diabetes Management? Patient information, Diabetes Clinical Research Unit of Mount Sinai Hospital Toronto for Sherwood Medical Industries Canada, Inc., distributed 1997.

What You Should Know About Aspartame. International Food Information Council, Washington, D.C., November 4, 1996.

What You Should Know About Humulin. Booklet, Eli Lilly of Canada, Inc., distributed 1997.

What You Should Know About MSG. International Food Information Council, Washington, D.C., September 1991.

What You Should Know About Sugars. International Food Information Council, Washington, D.C., May 1994.

Whitcomb, Randall. "The key to Type 2." *Diabetes Dialogue* (Vol. 43, No. 4), Winter 1996.

White, Jr., John R. "The pharmacologic management of patients with Type II diabetes mellitus in the era of new oral agents and insulin analogs." *Diabetes Spectrum* (Vol. 9, No. 4), 1996.

Willett, W. C., et al. "Intake of trans-fatty acids and risk of coronary heart disease among women." *Lancet* (Vol. 341), 1993:581–85.

Wormworth, Janice. "Toxins and tradition: The impact of food-chain contamination on the Inuit of northern Quebec." *Canadian Medical Association Journal* (Vol. 152, No. 8), April 15, 1995.

Yale, Jean-Francois. "Glucose results: Plasma or whole blood?" *Monitor* (Vol. 1, No. 2), MediSense Canada, Inc.

Yankova, Diliana. "Diabetes in Bulgaria." *Diabetes Dialogue* (Vol. 44, No. 1), Spring 1997.

"You are what you eat." *Equilibrium*, Canadian Diabetes Association (No. 1), 1996.

You Have Diabetes . . . Can You Have That? Booklet, Canadian Diabetes Association, 1995.

Your Blood Sugar Level . . . What Does It Tell You? Patient information, Eli Lilly of Canada, Inc., distributed 1997.

"Your diabetes healthcare team." *Equilibrium*, Canadian Diabetes Association (No. 1), 1996.

Your Kidneys. Patient information, Kidney Foundation of Canada, 1993.

Zinman, Bernard. "Insulin analogues." *Diabetes Dialogue* (Vol. 43, No. 4), Winter 1996.

Index